THIS JOURNAL BELONGS TO

_____

Moments and Milestones

Foreword
Introduction

Foreword

I**f there is one thing** I have learned from more than thirty years of teaching parents how to raise happy and successful children, it is that the quality of the parent-child relationship is the foundation on which all else is built. In fact, this is so important that current brain research is finding that the relationship between parent and child actually influences the physical development of the child's brain!

This critical relationship between parent and child begins in the mind of the parent, quite often the mother, at the moment she first wonders what it will be like to be a parent and what kind of parent she will be. An eight-year-old child playing with dolls and pretending to be a mommy is already developing a relationship with her future child. But nothing compares with the burst of energy and enthusiasm that is evoked with the knowledge that accompanies those two all-important words, "I'm pregnant." All the years of imagining are over and the reality that you will soon be a mother hits with a radiance that illuminates the critical role you are finally about to play in the cycle of life.

The relationship between you and your child takes a huge leap forward as the life inside you begins to grow and take shape. These months are not only about physical health—as important as that is—but also about attaching to your baby-to-be and starting to form the relationship that will govern so much of your future time together. One of the best ways to facilitate this bonding is to reflect on your experience during pregnancy through journaling. There is even some evidence that the act of writing down your thoughts and emotions can change your own neural pathways in ways that just thinking alone cannot. I am excited about this book and the power it has to deepen the bonding between you and your new child. I encourage you to take advantage of this opportunity to become an active parent-to-be and reflect, write, and act on the wisdom presented in these pages, wisdom that will unlock your own huge reservoirs of knowing how to build a strong and loving relationship with your child-to-be.

—Michael H. Popkin, Ph.D., Author, *Doc Pop's 52 Weeks of Active Parenting*

Dear Reader,

I just gave birth to my baby, so it is with great joy that I share with you, the expectant mother, this *Moments and Milestones Pregnancy Journal.*

Although this book gives you a heads-up on the key physical developments of your baby (the first day your baby's heart begins to beat; the day your baby can really hear your voice, and so on), most importantly, it will enable you to use these key developments as a springboard for exploring the physical and emotional journey *you* take during your pregnancy. The overall goal is to help you—through reflection and journaling—to feel not only enlightened but encouraged; not just to cope day by day while expecting your baby, but to experience deep joy and satisfaction!

What I discovered in my own pregnancy was that as I journaled on my feelings about my developing baby and the effect my pregnancy was having on me physically and emotionally, the better and happier I felt. Yes, I was grateful for those books that helped me understand the practical aspects of pregnancy, but I longed for a book that would not only help me know how my baby was developing but also allow me to explore my spiritual and emotional journey through the pregnancy. Although I searched the bookstores time and time again, there was no book to help me explore my changing emotional state; one that I knew was directly tied to my relationship with my baby. Through reflection and journaling I was better able to understand and use my emotional upheavals as a time for productive growth and change—and that made all the difference in my ability to care for myself and my unborn baby. I wanted to write the kind of journal that would help other women as my own journaling helped me. To make that a reality, I looked to my own mother, Bettie B. Youngs, not only because she is also a writer and gave me invaluable guidance in creating this journal, but also because we are close and it was natural for me to ask her about her own journey through her pregnancy with me.

This *Moments and Milestones Pregnancy Journal* will encourage you to actively explore your feelings about your pregnancy. It will strengthen the bond between you and your child even before your baby's birth, and it will prepare you for your baby's arrival. I believe you will find this book both useful and enriching.

Through each weekly entry you will be inspired to:

♡ Feel more positive and happy during this physically challenging time in your life

♡ Appreciate even more the wondrous miracle of creating and growing the life inside you—and fall in love with your child even before he or she is born

♡ Commit to the diet and lifestyle changes that will make you as healthy as possible during this critical time in your baby's development

♡ Learn more about the amazing stages of development as your child grows from a mere cluster of cells to a fully developed person

♡ Strengthen your relationship with your baby's father so that your child will enter the most loving and nurturing of homes

♡ Appreciate each milestone of these precious nine months in your life

One of the many special benefits of this book is that it can help you set the stage for a truly happy and healthy family life when your baby arrives. For example, if you have a poor or broken relationship with your mother or mother-in-law, questions in this journal can help you think about how to best mend fences, the goal being to foster the special and important bond between your new baby and his or her grandparents. This gives you a crucial opportunity to reach out and begin the process of improving this and other important relationships in your life.

Along with giving you an opportunity to record and reflect on the physical changes you are experiencing, each weekly affirmation will encourage you to address an emotional issue commonly faced by expectant mothers, such as:

♡ How can I love these nine months and see them as a gift?

♡ In what ways can I be supportive and encouraging to my partner to help him prepare for fatherhood?

♡ How can I help other family members—such as the baby's siblings or grandparents—prepare for welcoming this baby into the world?

♡ How will I handle the upcoming responsibilities of motherhood?

Each weekly entry will follow this format:

A Word to the Mother-to-Be. This personal message will directly address your point of view. This section will blend helpful information about what you may be experiencing physically or emotionally in any given week of pregnancy with updates about your baby's development and some of my own personal thoughts about what I was feeling during that particular week of *my* pregnancy. I'm hoping this section will make you feel as if you're chatting with your own expectant best friend.

This Week—BodyWise. This section begins the journal portion for each week. It will highlight the physical changes you can expect to go through in a particular week, such as morning sickness, the need for better nutrition, swelling of the hands and feet, and so forth, and then ask you to reflect on your body's own physical changes and needs. For instance, you will be prompted to reflect on questions about which methods you have found helpful in fighting nausea, how your new shape has affected your relationship with your partner, and what dietary changes you are making to support your hard-at-work body and your developing baby. Answering these questions will help guide you through a pregnancy that's healthy for both you and your baby.

This Week—SoulWise. Being pregnant may bring out an overwhelming array of feelings. Not only are your hormones affecting your emotions, but the significant changes in your life can also affect how you are feeling. It is not unusual for pregnant women to feel overjoyed at the prospect of motherhood while at the same time anxious about all the responsibilities this commitment entails. Pregnancy can also make you think about your life and priorities in a completely new way. This section will help you to examine your feelings about issues related to pregnancy and motherhood, as well as to other areas of your life, in light of your pregnancy. For example, weekly affirmations cover such topics as worries you have about your pregnancy and about impending motherhood, how your goals and priorities are changing now that you're expecting, your relationship with your own mother or with siblings, and ways in which you can be a loving and nurturing parent to your child. By reflecting and journaling on these and other topics related to your emotional and spiritual development, you can grow ever more positive and joyful as you prepare to welcome your child into the world.

Among This Week's Wonders. This section will outline some of the many wonders taking place as your baby takes shape and grows, following his or her progress from the first cluster of cells to a fully developed fetus ready to enter the world.

Three Things to Do This Week. In this section, you'll find one or two suggested to-do items along with space for adding one or two of your own. By following these short weekly lists, you can stay on track as you care for your own and your baby's well-being during your pregnancy and be better prepared for his or her arrival into your life and your home.

Bringing a child into the world is my greatest accomplishment to date, and I'm so glad that I have my own journal to remind me of this amazing time of my life. It is my hope that the *Moments and Milestones Pregnancy Journal* will give you the opportunity to reflect on and memorialize your own pregnancy, and that it will become a unique, important, and enriching book for you and your baby during your pregnancy. It is my prayer that through this book you will not only experience the same sense of awe and wonder I had throughout my own pregnancy, but be able to look back and clearly remember those feelings long after your baby is born.

Blessings and joy to you as you begin this wondrous adventure!

—Jennifer L. Youngs

Weeks 1 & 2

Preparing for Pregnancy

More so than almost any other event, becoming pregnant and preparing for motherhood will bring about great changes in your life.

A *Word to the Mother-to-Be:* During these two weeks, you are actually still in your pre-pregnancy stage. The beginning of your pregnancy is calculated from the start of your last menstrual period. This means that based on your doctor's computations, your pregnancy is counted for two weeks before it actually happens. This way of counting the weeks of pregnancy and fetal development is called the gestational age. Based on this system a full-term pregnancy is about 280 days, or 40 weeks. This contrasts with the ovulatory (or fertilization) age, which is counted from the day of conception. When tracking a pregnancy based on ovulatory age, a full-term pregnancy is thirty-eight weeks. Most medical professionals use gestational age to discuss pregnancy, and it is the system on which this book is based. Therefore, when you are in week 7 of pregnancy—and reading and journaling about week 7 in this book—you have been pregnant for five weeks, and when you are at week 20, you have been pregnant for eighteen weeks.

Although conception has not yet occurred, you can begin to prepare yourself body and soul for what lies ahead. You can also gather the resources needed for the physical and emotional changes you will experience throughout your pregnancy, so that you may face the next nine months with confidence and cherish all the milestones of this wondrous event in your life. Having this book means you are already off to a great start!

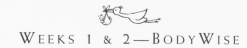

WEEKS 1 & 2—BODYWISE

At this time conception has not yet occurred. It will take place at the end of week 2, about midway between your menstrual cycles. Thus, if you have a 28-day cycle, ovulation will occur around day 14 following the start of your last menstrual cycle. Although you are not yet pregnant, it is important to prepare your body for the arduous work of nurturing a baby through nine months of development in your womb. Now is the time to develop healthy habits, such as eating a balanced and nutritious diet, giving up smoking and avoiding secondhand smoke, and abstaining from alcohol. It is also important at this time to begin taking prenatal vitamins. Folic acid should be started, if possible, three months *before* conception. (Many over-the-counter vitamins contain folic acid.) Of course, if your pregnancy is an unexpected surprise, it will not have been possible to spend these weeks preparing yourself for the pregnancy. So if you're reading this after the fact, think back on all the things you did that helped create an ideal environment for a developing baby. If you still have any concerns about things you should have done or not done, discuss these concerns with your doctor so that you can have peace of mind regarding your own and your baby's health, and so that you can learn the best ways possible to be ensure a healthy pregnancy.

In what ways was I prepared physically for becoming pregnant during these pre-pregnancy weeks, even though I may not have been consciously preparing to become pregnant?

_____

_____

_____

Which of my diet and lifestyle habits will be an advantage to me in preparation for the demands of pregnancy on my body?

_____

_____

Which of my diet and lifestyle habits are less than ideal for nurturing a baby? What changes will I make to eliminate these habits?

_____

_____

_____

WEEKS 1 & 2—SOULWISE

More so than almost any other event, becoming pregnant and looking forward to bringing a son or daughter into the world will bring about changes in your life. It will affect your priorities, your goals, and your plans for the future. Beginning from the day you find out that you are pregnant, all your choices and actions will be influenced by concern for your child. Whether you are considering how a particular action or choice will affect your developing baby's well-being or how it might have an impact on your family once your child is born, your perspective will certainly change in light of your new responsibility as an expectant parent. Taking time to reflect on and recognize some of the ways in which pregnancy and motherhood will affect you is a great way to prepare for the changes that await you.

What do I imagine will be the biggest change pregnancy will bring into my life? How can I prepare myself for this change?

_____

_____

_____

What do I imagine will be the biggest change motherhood will bring into my life? How can I prepare myself for this change?

_____

_____

_____

What is my greatest asset in my role as an expectant mom and in my future role as a parent?

_____

_____

_____

_____

_____

_____

AMONG THESE WEEKS' WONDERS:

1:

Your uterus sheds its lining through your period, and your hormones are preparing another egg for release.

2:

As the uterus sheds its lining, it prepares a lush new bed of blood-rich tissue for a fertilized egg and a growing fetus.

THREE THINGS TO DO IN WEEKS 1 & 2:

1. *Begin taking prenatal vitamins.*
2. *Develop a plan for healthy eating and a healthy lifestyle.*
3. _____

Week 3

The Miracle Begins!

From this moment on, the word love will take on

a brand-new meaning for you.

A *Word to the Mother-to-Be*: This week a miracle has occurred! On day 1 of this week, a single-cell organism was formed from the union of egg and sperm. And from that moment, a single cell will continue to develop, so that in nine months you will have a little child—a boy or a girl to love and nurture, to care for and teach about the wonders of the world.

It is difficult to comprehend what changes the new life forming within you will bring to your life. From this moment on, the words love and family will take on brand-new meanings for you. Open your heart to this experience and begin creating a happy and healthy life for your child.

Most likely, you're reading this entry when you're several weeks along in your pregnancy. So reading this entry in your journal is about thinking back and trying to remember the details about the week of this awesome moment. What day did conception occur? Were there any significant events going on in your life? As much as you can, recall all the important events of that week, so you can memorialize and celebrate this milestone in your life. Think about a special occasion you might have celebrated that week, special news you heard, and joyful times you experienced with family or friends.

WEEK 3 — BODYWISE

The instant I confirmed that I was pregnant, I retrieved my calendar and retraced everything I could about the first days of my pregnancy. I definitely wanted to determine the moment I conceived—the when and where—but I also wanted to retrace as much as I could about that week, especially about my activities during this time. I wanted to see all the happy events my baby had experienced with me—like the three days I had spent with a girlfriend visiting from out of town. I took delight in knowing that my baby had been a part of those joy-filled days!

What was the week of conception like for me? What was going on in my life?

_____

_____

_____

In the days following conception, did I intuitively know I was pregnant? What signs was I experiencing?

_____

_____

_____

What eating habits do I need to change to promote my baby's well-being? What is my plan for doing that?

_____

_____

_____

_____

Week 3—SoulWise

What feelings do you experience most intensely as you think about being pregnant? If you are currently feeling a confusing array of emotions—from surprised, happy, and ecstatic to fearful, worried, and anxious—it's all right! The one that matters most is confidence—confidence that you will do everything you can to nurture your baby and to celebrate this miracle in your life. So as you think back to the week you became pregnant when filling out these pages, also look forward. Focus on doing all you can to promote your baby's health in the weeks and months ahead.

How do I feel about being pregnant? Am I shocked, disappointed, elated, or worried? What are my most intense feelings?

_____

_____

_____

How is my partner feeling about learning that we are expecting? Have we discussed our feelings about becoming parents?

_____

_____

_____

In what ways do I feel I'll be a good parent to this baby?

_____

_____

_____

_____

Among This Week's Wonders:

Day 1:
Today, beginning with the moment of conception—the union of sperm and egg—a single-cell organism was formed.

Day 2:
The first cell division takes place. A two-sided ball is formed from the single-cell organism that was formed just yesterday.

Day 3:
The two identical cells have undergone additional cell divisions: two cells divided into four, four divided into eight, and then those eight became sixteen.

Day 4:
The sixteen-cell ball has traveled through your fallopian tube and enters your uterus.

Day 5:
The cell ball—now filled with fluid—divides into two groups. Those cells on the outside will become the placenta; those on the inside will form the baby.

Day 6:
The cell ball—now having multiplied into literally several hundred cells—attaches itself to your uterus so it can receive protection and needed oxygen and nutrients from your bloodstream.

Day 7:
Today the cell ball burrows into your uterine lining.

Three Things to Do This Week:

1. *Commit to doing all I can to care for this little life by taking care of my own health and well-being.*
2. *Review my diet and start eating more regularly and choosing healthier foods.*
3. _____

Week 4

Feeling a Little Emotional

Think about what you will do to prepare yourself—body and soul—to nurture your developing child.

A *Word to the Mother-to-Be*: During week 4, you were probably starting to feel some of the early symptoms of pregnancy, such as fatigue or nausea. It may have been during this week that you first realized that something about your body was different.

Most likely, you're reading week 4 after the fact. If so, use this opportunity to reflect on that time. Think about the first clues you may have had that you were pregnant. Think about ways in which you were creating a nurturing environment for your baby, even though you did not yet know you were expecting. Think about what else you will do to prepare yourself—body and soul—to nurture your developing child. Perhaps you need to reduce the stress in your life, to spend less time at work, or to mend a relationship. Or maybe your goal will be to focus more on your health—on eating well, avoiding unhealthy habits, and spending more time outdoors taking leisurely walks and enjoying nature. Now is the time to put into practice all those healthy ideals you may have been striving for. It's time to truly start caring for yourself, because by doing so you will also be caring for your baby.

WEEK 4—BODYWISE

You may not have realized it at the time, but your body was already working in high gear as your hormones revved up and the intricate work of your baby's development began. There were probably some signals—perhaps subtle, perhaps not—that your body was sending you at this time. Think about what those signals may have been. In retrospect, you may realize that some of those physical signs meant that your body was working overtime to support and sustain a developing baby. As you reflect on your second week, answer the following questions:

What physical signals was my body sending me this week that something big was going on? What did I attribute those signals to at the time?

_____

_____

_____

Did I notice any spotting ? Did I have any crampy feelings, like my period was going to start?

_____

_____

_____

Were my eating habits healthy in week 4? Which of my eating habits do I need to change?

_____

_____

_____

WEEK 4—SOULWISE

Although you may not have realized you were pregnant during week 4, you probably experienced some moods and feelings that left you wondering why you were suddenly so emotional. You may have found yourself going from a giggly mood to a teary-eyed one in a matter of minutes. Mood swings are normal during pregnancy, and are often more pronounced in the first trimester. One way to minimize them is to get plenty of rest and eat a healthy, balanced diet, taking care to keep your sugar and caffeine consumption to a minimum. Take time to recollect your moods and feelings from your week 4.

How was I feeling emotionally this week? Was I having mood swings for no reason?

_____

_____

_____

Did anyone comment on my moods? Did my partner or other family members say that I didn't seem my usual self during this time?

_____

_____

_____

Was I starting to wonder if I was pregnant? Was I hoping I was? What were my feelings about this possibility?

_____

_____

_____

What five words describe how I am feeling right now, as I think about my pregnancy?

_____

_____

_____

AMONG THIS WEEK'S WONDERS:

1:
The developing baby is now an embryo.

2:
The embryo will implant beneath the surface of the lining of the uterus.

3:
The amniotic sac forms (containing the amniotic fluid to sustain the developing baby).

4:
The yolk sac will appear (which will give rise to the baby's digestive tract).

5:
The placenta begins to form.

THREE THINGS TO DO THIS WEEK:

1. *Ask my doctor about prenatal vitamins if I haven't started taking them already.*
2. *Make changes in my hectic schedule to allow more time for rest and relaxation.*
3. _____

Week 5

Could I Be Pregnant?

Now is the time to truly put yourself—and your baby—first.

Be good to yourself and be good to your baby.

A **Word to the Mother-to-Be:** Like most expectant moms, by now you've probably missed a period and are starting to think that the way you've been feeling is more than just a case of the flu or a cold coming on. If you've been hoping to get pregnant, by now you may have already picked up a home pregnancy kit or are giving the possibility of pregnancy serious thought. For some women, however, this week can come and go without any extraordinary changes to alert them that they are pregnant. It may not be until the onset of severe morning sickness that the possibility of a pregnancy dawns on them or when a combination of symptoms makes the possibility unmistakable.

Whatever your particular circumstances, by week 5 the telltale symptoms have most likely gotten your attention! There is no mistaking the possibility that you're pregnant. Now is the time to truly put yourself—and your baby—first. It is time to make your own health and well-being a priority, to make plans to live a healthy lifestyle, to get plenty of rest, and to simply take time to enjoy the miracle happening inside you.

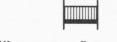

WEEK 5—BODYWISE

Your body is starting to send you some unmistakable signs of your pregnancy. Perhaps you've missed your period. If you weren't feeling breast tenderness or queasiness last week, you may be by now. You're probably asking yourself, "Should I buy the pregnancy test?" "Should I wait another week?" "Am I getting my hopes up for nothing?" Or perhaps even, "Did I goof up?" Think about the telltale signs of pregnancy you experienced during week 5.

Was this the week when I had my "aha!" moment—realizing that I was probably pregnant? What made me realize it?

_____

_____

_____

What new physical signs am I experiencing this week that weren't noticeable a week ago?

_____

_____

_____

Have my physical symptoms affected my relationship with my partner? For instance, have I been more interested in being intimate or less interested?

_____

_____

_____

🖉 *How can I take extra care of myself to alleviate some of the discomfort I am feeling and tend to the special needs my body has during this time?*

_____

_____

_____

WEEK 5—SOULWISE

The physical discomforts that you may be experiencing by this time can likely also affect your emotions. If you're feeling fatigued and nauseous, for example, chances are you're not in great spirits. Add the work of your hormones during this time and surely you are experiencing emotions that are more intense—and more unpredictable—than usual. Whatever your feelings at this point in your pregnancy, whether elation or frustration, realize that it's okay to experience many conflicting feelings at this stage. Be good to yourself, acknowledge any unpleasant emotions, and consider ways you will create a more peaceful, pleasant environment for yourself.

🖉 *What are some of the emotions I am experiencing at this time?*

_____

_____

_____

🖉 *How are my physical discomforts affecting my feelings about being pregnant? What am I doing to help myself feel better?*

_____

_____

_____

Is my partner supportive? Is he sympathetic to my physical discomfort and my emotional sensitivity? How can I help him to understand how I feel?

_____

_____

_____

AMONG THIS WEEK'S WONDERS:

1:
It is now possible to identify the baby's head and tail.

2:
The baby's first blood cells are formed.

3:
The cells now are so complete that a genetic blueprint exists within each one telling it what to do and orders its migration to the spot in the developing body where it will create specific organs.

4:
The vertebrae—the bones of the spine—begin to form.

5:
The baby's primitive heart forms and begins working to move around the oxygen and nutrient-rich blood cells that will feed the developing tissues.

THREE THINGS TO DO THIS WEEK:

1. *Make a conscious effort to eat a healthy diet, drink plenty of fluids, and get extra rest.*
2. *Avoid people and situations that create stress in my life.*
3. _____

Week 6

Keeping My Baby Safe

The tiny baby inside of you—smaller than a grain of rice

right now—already has a little heart.

A Word to the Mother-to-Be: Among the many things happening to your developing baby this week is the marvel of a little heart that miraculously starts beating! The tiny baby inside of you—smaller than a grain of rice right now—already has a little heart. What an amazing thought! Eyes, arms, and a brain are also beginning to form. As your baby grows, he is becoming more dependent on you for healthy development. He eats what you eat. He drinks what you drink. He breathes what you breathe. Your baby's growing parts need lots of nutrients.

On the day that I learned that my child's heart had begun to beat, my life changed. From that point on, nothing was more important to me than protecting my unborn child. Of course, I still worried about whether I had done anything to harm my child—had I been around secondhand smoke before I was aware I was pregnant? Have I been eating properly? I carefully thought about the preceding three weeks so that I might discuss with my doctor any concerns I had. You may want to do the same thing now. Then commit yourself fully to caring for yourself and your baby.

WEEK 6—BODYWISE

By now, you're probably imagining what you'll look like pregnant. If you're like me, you've already been checking out your profile in the mirror—although it probably hasn't changed. At this point, aside from a certain glow that may leave your friends and family wondering, your pregnancy will still be a well-kept secret. Think about your changing body as you respond to the following journal questions:

What do I perceive to be the most visible sign of my pregnancy? How do I feel about this change?

_____

_____

_____

Am I eating well enough and taking the right vitamin supplements to support my baby? If not, what changes will I make starting now?

_____

_____

_____

Does the thought that my child now has a heart make him feel more real? Have I tried to imagine it beating along with mine?

_____

_____

_____

WEEK 6—SOULWISE

As the saying goes, having a baby changes everything. One of the changes a new baby will bring, especially a first baby, is the amount of time you and your partner spend together, and how you spend it. The birth of a child can cause hurt feelings and conflict as the demands of a newborn and the need to spend quality time as a couple compete for a new mom's time. Now is the time to strengthen your relationship. Arrange to spend time alone with your husband, plan special outings, and build your communication skills to reduce any stress to your relationship that a newborn may cause.

Does my partner share my excitement about the pregnancy? Does he have any concerns I need to be sensitive to and address?

_____

_____

_____

Do my partner and I have a strong relationship? How can we enrich and nurture our relationship over the next eight months?

_____

_____

_____

Does being pregnant make me anxious about being intimate? Have I talked to my doctor about my concerns about sexual activity during my pregnancy?

_____

_____

_____

Which of my partner's qualities and personality traits am I most grateful for? Do I tell him so often enough?

_____

_____

AMONG THIS WEEK'S WONDERS:

1:
This week your baby's heart begins to beat!

2:
This week, the collection of cells transforms into an oblong body.

3:
Brain cells and the spinal cord begin to form.

4:
Nerve cells—those that will govern bodily functions and spark consciousness—are formed.

5:
The outer layer encloses the baby's torso.

6:
Arm buds appear.

7:
Eyes are beginning to form.

THREE THINGS TO DO THIS WEEK:

1. *Go to the library or bookstore and pick up a pregnancy guide.*
2. *Learn as much as I can about the ways in which my baby is developing this week, and the changes that he went through before I even knew I was pregnant.*
3. _____

Week 7

Seeing the World in a Whole New Way

Take time to recognize the gifts you bring to

the task of motherhood.

A *Word to the Mother-to-Be:* For me, week 7 was a time of mixed emotions. My husband and I had definitely not planned this pregnancy, so I found myself worrying about whether I had done everything right before I became pregnant and during the early weeks of my pregnancy—before I had confirmed my pregnancy. Because I hadn't prepared myself physically—with the proper nutrition, sufficient rest, and prenatal vitamins—I worried about whether everything was okay with my developing baby. But then came the sheer elation that I was going to have a baby!

Suddenly, when I looked in the mirror, I saw myself in a whole new light—and the whole world looked different as well. Now, everywhere I looked I saw babies, pregnant women, and baby things—clothes, strollers, toys, and all sorts of baby accoutrements.

By this time in your pregnancy, you probably know just what I mean. As your child continues to grow, so does your excitement.

As you think about all the joys and responsibilities of caring for your child, make a commitment to care for your own health and well-being. Focus on the nutritional needs of you and your baby. Talk to your doctor and review a pregnancy guide to be sure you are providing your child with the nutrition she needs. Cherish your pregnancy by making your health and that of your baby your number-one priority.

WEEK 7 — BODYWISE

By week 7, you've probably confirmed your due date with your doctor, making the idea of being pregnant feel all the more real. In addition, by this point in your pregnancy you are likely to be experiencing more symptoms. Some of the most common symptoms include fatigue and sleepiness, a frequent need to urinate, heartburn, and food cravings or aversions. You have probably started to notice that your clothes are getting a little tight around the waist and chest. As the signs of pregnancy become more distinct, you probably feel more and more eager to share the news with friends and family members.

What are some distinct physical symptoms I'm feeling that are either definitely or likely to be related to being pregnant?

_____

_____

_____

What foods am I craving? What foods can I suddenly not tolerate even the smell of? What are the most dramatic changes to my food preferences?

_____

_____

_____

If I normally engage in strenuous physical activity, how much should I cut back during my pregnancy? Have I discussed this issue with my doctor?

_____

_____

_____

Week 7—SoulWise

By week 7, your emotions may be becoming somewhat unpredictable. You might find yourself going from giddy to sad in a matter of minutes and for no apparent reason. In addition to the hormonal changes affecting your moods, you are likely to be feeling physically tired, or even fatigued, making you even more sensitive. Even if you were a rock before—rarely letting others see you cry—you may suddenly find yourself ready to cry over a sappy television show, or when you can't find your car keys, or for no reason at all. At times, the weight of being responsible for another human being—not just for the next seven and a half months, but for many years after that—may seem daunting. Rest assured that these changing emotions are a natural part of being pregnant. When you start to feel anxious, take time to recognize your gifts and abilities that will enable you to nurture your unborn baby and to be a capable and loving parent to your child when she is born.

What emotions or mood swings have caught me by surprise this week? What emotions am I feeling at the thought that I am responsible for the health and welfare of my unborn child?

_____

_____

_____

_____

What special gifts do I bring to the task of motherhood?

_____

_____

_____

Among This Week's Wonders:

1:
The size of your baby doubles this week.

2:
Your baby's blood is circulating, distributing nutrition and oxygen to all the tiny developing organs.

3:
Facial features begin to form—the chin, cheeks, upper jaw, eyes, ears, nose, mouth, nostrils, voice box (larynx), and windpipe (trachea).

4:
The chest and abdominal cavities continue to form.

5:
Lung buds appear.

6:
The outer layer of skin encloses the torso.

7:
Skull bones begin to fuse.

Three Things to Do This Week:

1. *Get plenty of rest and pamper myself.*
2. _____
3. _____

Week 8

Being Sick, but Staying Fit

When morning sickness seems to be getting the best of you, do your best to get the most nutrition out of every bite you eat.

A Word to the Mother-to-Be: By the time week 8 rolls around, you have probably grown accustomed to dealing with morning sickness. As you may have discovered by now, that name is more than a little misleading, because morning sickness is not limited to the morning but can strike at any time. Just as I began to feel aglow because of my pregnancy, I was struck with intense morning sickness that left me feeling anything but glowing. Of course, morning sickness doesn't affect all pregnant women. I have talked to women who tell me they didn't experience even one day of nausea! If you aren't one of those lucky ones, however, you'll need to figure out ways to combat nausea. In my case, I found that eating smaller meals helped. I also took my prenatal vitamins in the evening because that made me feel less queasy. Some women I know found that sucking on a slice of lemon was a great way to alleviate nausea. Figure out what works for you, discuss with your doctor ways to ensure that you and your baby are getting the proper nutrition, and remember that this will not last through your whole pregnancy.

WEEK 8—BODYWISE

Although you may be experiencing morning sickness, do your best to take in enough nutrition. Choose your foods carefully to avoid nausea and to get the most nutrition out of every snack or meal. And if you find yourself experiencing intense food cravings or aversions, be sure that heeding them isn't causing you to fill up on empty calories or to deprive you and your baby of essential nutrients. If you find that you are craving brownies and ice cream, for example, consider making that only an occasional treat and finding a healthier way to satisfy your craving. If the sight of spinach suddenly repels you, be sure that you are eating enough leafy greens in another form. Sometimes the iron in prenatal vitamins can cause nausea. If this happens to you, speak to your doctor. Most of all, if nausea is keeping you from eating as much as you should, try to relax and aim for quality rather than quantity. Your baby doesn't need a ton of food right now, but he does need the best food for his growth and development.

How am I feeling this week? What physical changes am I experiencing?

_____

_____

_____

If I am feeling nauseous, what strategies do I have for feeling better? Which foods are easiest on my stomach?

_____

_____

_____

What concerns or questions do I have that I would like to discuss with my doctor?

_____

_____

_____

_____

What foods that I am craving do I need to consume in limited quantities? What foods should I make a greater effort to include in my diet?

_____

_____

WEEK 8 — SOULWISE

Being pregnant is generally a joyous experience. But every woman who has gone through the experience can tell you that it's not always smooth sailing. Whether the culprit is morning sickness or hormonal fluctuations, you are bound to have some trying days. But you can always take steps to minimize the negative physical aspects of pregnancy. For example, when it comes to morning sickness, once you get to know the foods or smells that set you off, you can be careful to avoid them. Feeling better physically will help you to feel better emotionally. Also, avoid situations (or people) that tend to make you edgy. Do whatever you can to create a pleasant atmosphere for yourself, one that will enhance your overall sense of well-being.

Have my hormones made my moods a bit unpredictable? Does knowing that pregnancy causes my mood swings help me to deal with them?

_____

_____

My best day this week has been:

_____

_____

My worst day was:

_____

_____

✎ *What are some things I can do to ensure that my environment—the people and situations around me—will help me keep a positive attitude?*

_____

_____

AMONG THIS WEEK'S WONDERS:

1:
The area of the brain that coordinates muscle development begins to develop.

2:
Jaw and face muscles are beginning to form.

3:
The kidneys are formed and begin to produce urine.

4:
The tissue that will form the hands and fingers appears.

5:
The baby's legs now resemble paddles.

6:
The intestines are beginning to form within the umbilical cord.

7:
Pigment within the baby's retina will be present this week.

THREE THINGS TO DO THIS WEEK:

1. *Commit to avoiding situations or people that cause me to feel tense or stressed.*
2. *Talk to my doctor about managing any nausea I'm experiencing and ways to ensure I'm getting the nutrients my baby needs.*
3. _____

Week 9

Sweet Anticipation!

*Focus on the gift that your child is to you and the blessings
she will bring into your life.*

A Word to the Mother-to-Be: By now you're no doubt beginning to feel your body change, not only in relationship to the fact that you're pregnant but in preparation for the coming baby. Your breasts are swelling and feel tender to the touch. Your uterus is now approximately the size of an orange. No doubt, too, your thoughts are constantly turning to the baby you are carrying. You may be wondering about the gender, what the baby will look like—will she have your eyes? her father's nose?—and how her first smile will make you feel. As you think ahead to the time following your baby's birth, also think about all the wonderful things going on now. This week, the baby's organs have already formed, and her bones are beginning to form as well. All this while she still measures just over 1 inch! Even though you may sometimes feel like you can hardly wait to hold your newborn baby, there are so many joys and wonders along the way. Take time to savor them all and to appreciate their wonder.

WEEK 9—BODYWISE

It is important during your baby's early development that you stay as healthy as possible. Serious illness in the mother can cause harm to the baby, so guard your health by avoiding people who have a contagious illness, such as a cold or a stomach virus; wash your hands frequently; and maintain healthy eating habits to keep your immune system strong. This doesn't mean you should panic if you come down with a cold, but see your doctor if you think you might be coming down with something or were in the company of someone who is ill.

Have I had any illnesses since my baby's conception? If so, did I discuss them with my doctor?

_____

_____

_____

What steps am I taking to stay healthy and to maintain a strong immune system? Am I eating well and getting enough rest to support the needs and demands of my pregnancy?

_____

_____

_____

Have I told my partner of the precautions I'm taking to avoid getting sick during my pregnancy and asked him to take extra precautions, too?

_____

_____

_____

Am I comfortable avoiding certain social situations that may put me at risk of getting sick? Will I be overly concerned about hurting other people's feelings? Do I need to feel more comfortable asserting myself for my child's well-being?

_____

_____

_____

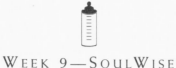

WEEK 9—SOULWISE

As you start thinking about your child and what she will be like—will she be smart? will she be outgoing or shy? will she be like you, or like her father? will she be healthy?—think also about how much you'll love your child, regardless of the color of her hair, her talents, or who she looks like. Focus on the gift that your child is to you and the blessings she will bring into your life. Know that no matter what, you will love your child with all your heart and will care for her and nurture her with a loving heart.

What are my hopes for this baby? Will I love my child and know that she is a blessing in my life no matter what?

_____

_____

_____

What are the most important things I want for my child right now?

_____

_____

_____

What are the most important things I want for my child after she is born?

_____

_____

_____

Among This Week's Wonders:

1:
This week, your baby will be four times as long as she was a month ago!

2:
Cartilage and bone are beginning to form.

3:
The elbows are visible, and the baby's legs are now at their proper location and proportional size for this stage of development.

4:
The nasal opening and the tip of the baby's nose are formed.

5:
The baby's arms now bend at the elbow.

6:
Hairs begin to develop.

Three Things to Do This Week:

1. *Take a break from life's busyness and enjoy some quiet time for reflection.*
2. _____
3. _____

Week 10

It's a Beautiful World!

Don't let needless worry diminish your enjoyment

of this special time in your life.

A *Word to the Mother-to-Be:* When I read about the forming of my baby's little eyes this week, it made me think about the precious work I was doing—the magnificent undertaking of doing everything I could to help him be as healthy and perfect as possible. And just thinking about the wonder of his eyes forming made me thankful for my own ability to see the beauty of the world around me. Suddenly, I was more aware of all there was to see—the clouds, the flowers, the smiles on people's faces. It was as if I were noticing these things for the first time.

By week 10, you are fully in the throes of pregnancy. You surely feel pregnant by this time, and may even be starting to look pregnant. By now, there is also a lot going on with your baby. Along with his developing eyes, your baby has a beating heart and arms and legs with the beginnings of fingers and toes. His external ears are completely formed, as is the upper lip. There is certainly a lot to think about and a lot to feel excited about.

WEEK 10—BODYWISE

Although others may not notice that you're pregnant, by now you can probably see some changes in your appearance. The pigmentation changes that accompany pregnancy may begin to show. For example, your nipples may be darkening or your skin may look blotchy. You may notice a rounding to your tummy and feel the need to leave the top button on your pants undone. When you look in the mirror, you may notice that you look just a little fuller around the waist and chest. Your face, too, might be starting to look a little fuller, prompting comments such as, "I don't know what you've done, but you sure look good." Also common at this stage of pregnancy are headaches, frequently caused by hormonal changes, fatigue, tension, or hunger. If you find yourself suddenly experiencing frequent headaches, try to determine the cause—for example, you may notice that your headaches typically follow delays between meals or snacks—then do your best to eliminate the causes. Although you should be avoiding pain relievers, talk to your doctor about what, if any, over-the-counter remedies are okay to use when you just need to take something.

Is my stomach looking rounder these days? Do I feel the need to wear looser clothes or unbutton the top button of my pants?

_____

_____

_____

What are the most distinct physical changes I've experienced up to this point in my pregnancy? What in my opinion is the most dramatic change?

_____

_____

_____

Have I been experiencing frequent headaches? If so, what seems to provoke them? What can I do to eliminate some of the causes of my headaches?

_____

_____

_____

Week 10—SoulWise

Some women are surprised at the number of worries that accompany pregnancy. They worry that their baby isn't developing properly, that they might have harmed the baby by something they consumed, that they'll never lose their baby fat, that their marriage will never be the same, that they'll be confined to bed rest, and on it goes. Do you find yourself worrying about similar or other matters? Of course, as an expectant mom you want to do everything you can to ensure the health and well-being of your baby, but beyond doing everything in your power, you simply need to surrender worry over the things you can't control. If you make a conscious effort to banish worry from your mind—and to trust that all will be taken care of—you'll be surprised at how much more lighthearted you'll feel and how much more you'll enjoy your pregnancy as a truly special time in your life.

Some issues that I've been worrying about lately include the following:

_____

_____

_____

Of these, the ones I can control are:

_____

_____

_____

Some issues over which I have no control but have been feeling some anxiety are the following:

_____

_____

_____

Among This Week's Wonders:

1:
Your baby's brain is starting to look human as lines and fissures form on its surface.

2:
A baby girl's clitoris begins to form, and a boy's scrotum starts to swell.

3:
The retina of the baby's eyes is now fully pigmented. Your baby has eye color!

4:
The external ears have finished developing.

5:
Baby is getting taste buds!

6:
The tail has disappeared.

Three Things to Do This Week:

1. *Take pictures of my new shape and start an album for weekly or monthly snapshots showing off my growing form!*
2. *Make a shopping list of the new clothes I'll need to accommodate my new body.*
3. _____

Week 11

Extra! Extra!

*Now may be the time to share the news . . . and
to enjoy the special treatment you'll start getting.*

A *Word to the Mother-to-Be:* This is a big week for your little baby. The developments that will have taken place by week 11 include the preliminary functioning of the internal organs—for example, the kidneys now produce urine and the stomach produces gastric juices. Also by week 11, the rapid steady beat of the baby's heart can be seen with a sonogram. If you've already had your first sonogram—as I did during week 11—then you've not only had a sneak preview of your baby but a chance to see and hear her little heart beat.

Of course, other amazing things are going on as well. For instance, your baby's newly developing legs, arms, and hands are beginning to move around. Ever more a little person, your baby now has facial expressions, which could be similar to yours!

By now you've probably divulged the news about your pregnancy or are ready to do so. Letting others in on your exciting news will ensure that your family and friends will be sympathetic to your aches, pains, and fatigue. Chances are it will also mean that the people around you will be just a little more accommodating—maybe letting you off the hook on after-dinner clean-up or giving you time to just sit and rest. When this happens, graciously and gratefully accept it, and take advantage of the opportunity to work a little less and rest a little more. Bringing a baby into the world is no easy task—accept the help you're offered.

WEEK 11 — BODYWISE

Just think about all that is happening inside you right now as your baby grows. No wonder your body is exhausted! You may not look very pregnant yet, but your body feels otherwise! Take the tiredness as a cue that you should get some rest and extra sleep. It's not uncommon to have sleep problems at this stage, even if you've never had trouble sleeping before. If you're experiencing mild insomnia, it is likely because your mind is racing, thinking about your baby as she is developing and anticipating the changes she'll bring into your life in just a few months. If you're having trouble sleeping, some simple things you can do to get a better night's sleep include getting more exercise in the daytime (talk to your doctor about suitable exercise, and don't work out too close to bedtime), developing a bedtime routine that will promote relaxation, or simply staying up just a little bit later.

Am I having trouble sleeping at night? What seems to be keeping me from sleeping through the night? What can I do about it?

_____

_____

_____

Have I asked my partner to lend an extra hand in ways that he can?

_____

_____

Do I try to be Super Pregnant Woman or am I realistic in my expectations of myself during my pregnancy? What adjustments do I have to make?

_____

_____

_____

Week 11—SoulWise

Like most pregnant women, you probably spend quite a bit of time daydreaming about what your child will look like and what sort of personality she will have. Will she be laid back or feisty? Will she be like you or like her father, or a perfect combination of the two of you? Of course, you've probably also started to think about what will be the perfect name for your child—one that will truly capture her personality.

When I daydream about my baby, I imagine her having the following personality traits:

_____

_____

_____

What personality traits do I most want my baby to have? Why?

_____

_____

_____

Do the baby's father and I agree on names? (If you haven't decided, you can list possible names on pages 169–170 of the "Planning for Baby" section.)

_____

_____

_____

Among This Week's Wonders:

1:
The baby's head makes up more than half of her length.

2:
Fingernails, toenails, and hair follicles will appear.

3:
The arms and hands are forming; individual fingers are just barely discernible.

4:
The backbone houses the spinal cord from which nerve fibers
extend into the rest of the body.

5:
Many of the baby's organs have already begun to function. The kidneys
produce urine, and the stomach produces gastric juice.

6:
The baby has begun to move: The first visible motion is the rapid steady
beating of the heart, but soon small bodily movements show that
nerve impulses coming from the brain are instructing muscles to contract.

7:
The baby's irises are developing.

Three Things to Do This Week:

1. *Get used to accepting other people's accommodating treatment toward me, and learn to accept it graciously.*
2. *Start a list of favorite names and the special meanings they have for me and my partner (you can use pages 169-170 of this book to list possible names).*
3. _____

Week 12

Sharing the Joys and Worries

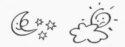

Sharing your feelings will increase your happiness

and diminish your worries.

A *Word to the Mother-to-Be:* For me, week 12 was a real turning point in the way I felt. The nausea began subsiding, and the "feeling good" times began moving in. Thank goodness, too. I was really very sick and tired of feeling, well, sick and tired! Many women who have experienced morning sickness find that around week 12 those symptoms begin to subside. When that happens, you can begin to feel more comfortable and better able to focus on all the great things that are going on in your baby's development. By week 12, your baby measures about 2½ to 3 inches, and his circulatory and urinary systems are operating. His tiny fingernails are forming, and the bony part of his palate has finished forming. For me, knowing all the changes that were taking place from week to week and month to month, both with my baby and my own body, was exciting as well as fun for me and my husband to keep track of together. If you haven't already done so, get a good pregnancy guide that can help you keep track of your baby's development.

WEEK 12—BODYWISE

As morning sickness starts to subside, you may find yourself with an increased appetite. This, of course, is a good thing, especially if you've had intense nausea that has kept you from eating the variety and quantity of foods that you need. But with your increased appetite might come an increased worry about weight gain. Clearly, pregnancy is not the time to be watching your weight. You have an increased appetite for a very good reason: You are eating for two. You need to take in enough nutrition to sustain your own body as well as to accommodate the growth of your child into a healthy newborn. However, you may wonder how much is too much? Medical experts generally agree that weight gain in the 25- to 35-pound range is ideal. On average, very little of that is gained in the first trimester—only 3 or 4 pounds. If you find yourself gaining weight too quickly, you might want to evaluate the quality of what you are eating, rather than the quantity. Most important, watch what you eat, but don't diet. Talk to your doctor about your concerns regarding weight gain and get his or her advice about choosing the foods that are right for you and your baby.

How much weight have I gained so far? Am I eating foods that are healthy and high in nutrition?

_____

_____

_____

What advice has my doctor given me regarding proper nutrition and weight gain?

_____

_____

_____

Foods I need to eat more of include:

_____

_____

_____

Foods that I like but know I should avoid include:

_____

_____

_____

Week 12 — SoulWise

If you've experienced a miscarriage in the past, you may still be afraid to get your hopes up in case things don't work out. But now is the time to put things into perspective. Miscarriages most commonly occur in the first trimester, and you have just about concluded that phase of your pregnancy. Know that the great majority of women who experience a miscarriage go on to have healthy pregnancies. So if you're feeling anxious because of an earlier miscarriage, remember that you are not alone. Share your worries with other women. Also, remember that countless women who suffer through miscarriages go on to have healthy babies. Rely on your faith to see you through the days ahead.

Have any of my friends or family members experienced a miscarriage? Do they have children now? Can I talk to them about my concerns?

_____

_____

_____

If I've experienced a miscarriage or difficult pregnancy in the past, how has it affected my feelings about this pregnancy?

_____

_____

In what ways has being pregnant made me I happier than I've ever been?

_____

_____

_____

Among This Week's Wonders:

1:
Your baby is starting to get fingernails.

2:
The baby's gall bladder, pancreas, and thyroid will finish developing.

3:
The muscles in your baby's digestive tract will start working. Even though he's not moving food through it now, he's making practice moves.

4:
The bony part of your baby's palate finishes forming.

5:
Tooth buds are appearing.

Three Things to Do This Week:

1. _Expand my wardrobe to include looser and more comfortable clothing._

2. _____

3. _____

Week 13

Taking a Personal Inventory

Being pregnant is a great reason to examine your priorities.

A *Word to the Mother-to-Be:* Being pregnant is a great reason to take a personal inventory—to think about your life, your accomplishments, and your plans for the future. If you haven't already begun this process, now is a great time to start. Especially if you're going to be a parent for the first time, this child will definitely take you on a new path in life. You may have to adjust or postpone goals you've made. In their place, you might choose entirely new goals, ones that are more focused on your child and the ways in which you would like to be the best parent possible to her.

There is a lot to think about as you look forward to your role as a parent. During my pregnancy, I thought about how much I genuinely wanted to be a good mother. I wanted to do the right things and to be a good role model for my child. I thought about the values I wanted to impart to her, and the loving environment in which I wanted her to be raised. I thought about how I wanted my child to grow up looking up to me and being proud of me. I also thought about the way my own parents lived their lives and the sacrifices they'd made for me, and knew that my husband and I would also be making sacrifices for our child, because of our love for her. As parents, I knew that our highest priority would always be our child.

WEEK 13 — BodyWise

By week 13, as your belly starts to show unmistakable signs of your pregnancy, you may be starting to fret about stretch marks and looking for ways to prevent them. Ninety percent of pregnant women develop stretch marks during pregnancy, typically on the breasts, abdomen, and hips. However, there are certain things you can do to improve your odds of avoiding them. First, remember that moderate, gradual weight gain is less likely to result in stretch marks. Also, maintaining a healthy diet and drinking plenty of fluids can promote your skin's elasticity and reduce the extent to which you'll get stretch marks. Finally, remember that fancy creams that promise to help you avoid stretch marks probably won't keep that promise. But go ahead and use them if you like—at the very least they'll keep your skin moisturized.

Am I concerned that I will get stretch marks? What other lasting physical changes to my body do I worry about?

_____

_____

_____

What can I do to keep myself in the best possible shape during my pregnancy in a way that will not be harmful to my baby? For example, should I be drinking more fluids, getting more light exercise?

_____

_____

_____

This week I will pamper myself by doing the following:

_____

_____

WEEK 13—SoulWise

Being pregnant prompted me to take inventory of my life. It made me want to be the best person I could be. I wanted to be a good role model, and to be the kind of person my child would always be proud of. The time during which you're anticipating becoming a parent is a great opportunity to reevaluate your life, to reconsider your goals and priorities, to grow stronger in your faith, and to think about ways in which you'd like to be a better person. If you aspire to be more generous, to make peace with a family member with whom you've had a falling out, to build better relations with your parents or siblings, now is a great time to make those ideals a reality, because by enriching your own life you will also be enriching the life you will share with your child.

What qualities do I have that will make me a good mother?

_____

_____

_____

Do I have any goals for myself that I now feel an urgency to fulfill? What are these goals, and how can I begin to reach them?

_____

_____

_____

In what ways have I already begun to adjust my priorities?

_____

_____

_____

1:

This week or the next, your baby's kidneys will begin to
excrete urine into the amniotic fluid.

2:

Baby's intestines are moving from the umbilical cord to their proper place
in the body where they will continue their development.

3:

Baby's vocal cords are formed.

4:

Twenty baby teeth form in baby's gums.

5:

The baby's liver starts to release bile.

THREE THINGS TO DO THIS WEEK:

1. *Set three self-improvement goals for myself.*
2. *Call or write my mother to let her know all the ways she was a good mother to me.*
3. _____

Week 14

Celebrating the End of the First Trimester

Whether you have a son or a daughter, you will have

the child who is perfect for you.

A *Word to the Mother-to-Be:* Week 14 brings you to the start of your fourth month of pregnancy and your second trimester. By now your baby, now called a fetus, is just over 3 inches long. More internal organs are developing, the circulatory and urinary systems are operating, and the liver produces bile. By now, too, reproductive organs have developed, and your baby's gender can probably be identified in a sonogram. During my sonogram in my fourteenth week, my doctor told me she was 90 percent certain that my little baby was a girl. Wow! My baby was a she—a daughter! Knowing this made my thoughts of motherhood seem so much more real. I discarded my list of possible boys' names, and began naming my daughter. Now I could refer to her by name. Of course, her name changed on an almost daily basis, but it was still exciting to have a name for my daughter. Now I could say, "Kendahl, mommy loves you" or "Brooke, what shall we have for lunch today?"

WEEK 14—BODYWISE

Heartburn and indigestion seemed to be my constant companions during my pregnancy—not an uncommon problem in pregnancy. Although typically indigestion can be caused by overeating, during pregnancy it is more likely caused by the increased amounts of progesterone and estrogen your body produces, which result in the relaxation of smooth muscle tissue, including that of the gastrointestinal tract. Frequent heartburn during pregnancy is also caused by the relaxing effect of hormones on muscle tissue. In this case, the sphincter muscle between the stomach and the esophagus relaxes, allowing stomach acid and food to back up into the esophagus.

Simple things you can do to reduce the frequency of indigestion and heartburn include, for example, eating smaller, more frequent meals; eating slowly; not wearing clothing that is snug around the waist; and avoiding highly seasoned foods. Although you won't be free of these symptoms anytime soon, you can be relieved that you're past your first trimester, because now you'll be entering a somewhat easier phase in your pregnancy. The second trimester is typically the easiest on the expectant mom, with fewer discomforts and less fatigue than in the first or third trimesters.

How have I changed my eating habits to lessen the chances of digestive difficulties?

_____

_____

_____

What foods seem to be the easiest on my stomach? Which foods make me the most uncomfortable?

_____

_____

_____

Have I noticed any difference yet in the way I feel now that I'm through with the first trimester?

_____

_____

WEEK 14—SoulWise

Any day now, you'll be able to find out your baby's sex if you wish. Most expectant parents say, of course, that they don't care whether the baby is a boy or a girl, as long as the baby is healthy. And certainly that's true. But, even so, deep down inside we often picture ourselves with either a boy or a girl. Perhaps you see yourself braiding your daughter's hair, giving her a favorite doll you've saved from your own childhood, and getting her a canopy bed. Or maybe you can more easily picture yourself teaching a son how to bat a ball, drawing pictures with him, and playing in the park. But in the end, whether we picture ourselves with a son or a daughter, it always turns out that we have the child who is perfect for us and whom we will love with our whole heart.

Deep down, am I hoping I'll have a boy or a girl? What are my partner's hopes?

_____

_____

If I have a girl, what dreams do I have for her? What activities do I want to share with her?

_____

_____

_____

If I have a boy, what dreams do I have for him? What activities do I want to share with him?

_____

_____

_____

Among This Week's Wonders:

1:
Baby is developing an opposable thumb! All of his fingers are beginning to function.

2:
The baby's external sex organs are becoming visible. (You'll be able to tell if you're having a boy or a girl.)

3:
Baby practices breathing, even though he is breathing amniotic fluid in and out of his lungs instead of air.

4:
The spleen begins to function.

5:
Baby's salivary glands start working.

6:
The doctor can use a Doppler device to hear the baby's heartbeat.

7:
Your baby weighs between 1 to 2 ounces and is just over 3 inches long.

Three Things to Do This Week:

1. *Write a letter to my baby describing my feelings about having a son or a daughter.*
2. _____
3. _____

Week 15

Dealing with Unsolicited Advice

Don't let unsolicited advice or other people's lack of support dampen your joy.

A *Word to the Mother-to-Be:* At this point in your pregnancy, most of your family, friends, and even coworkers probably know that you're expecting. Letting others in on your news can be a wonderful thing, especially in the case of close friends and family members who will be anticipating your child's birth with excitement. It is also nice to get special treatment—a little extra rest, the more comfortable seat, specially prepared food—in deference to your "condition." However, you may not always enjoy the special attention you get. Pregnant women frequently complain about—and resent—all the unsolicited advice they receive. Whether this advice is from a mother, mother-in-law, friend who has kids who feels you can greatly benefit from her expertise, or coworker who just can't help but tell you what you should and shouldn't be eating, you're sure to find yourself on the receiving end of a great deal of well-intentioned but unwanted advice.

Dealing with this can be tricky. You don't want to upset people who genuinely care about you, but you do want to tell them that if you want advice from them, you'll ask for it. One way to deal with this pesky issue is to politely but firmly tell well-meaning people who give you unwanted advice that you've got a great pregnancy guide that you refer to for all sorts of pregnancy questions, and that you have a great doctor whom you really trust.

WEEK 15—BODYWISE

Your body will start undergoing more dramatic changes to accommodate the growing size of your baby. For instance, your uterus will begin to rise, and you may start to notice some swelling of your ankles and feet, and possibly even of your hands and face. The good news is that your breasts may be less tender than they were in the first trimester. You may also be experiencing somewhat less fatigue, and the worst of the morning sickness is likely to be over—which of course means you can now eat a greater variety of foods. By week 15, you are likely to be feeling better than you've felt in the preceding weeks of your pregnancy. Enjoy the change, but don't assume that you will now have boundless strength and energy. Continue to get plenty of rest and to eat well and frequently.

How am I feeling this week?

_____

_____

_____

Am I starting to notice more physical evidence of my pregnancy? What body changes have I noticed most recently?

_____

_____

Has anyone else commented on the changes they've seen in me? What was the nicest thing someone said?

_____

_____

_____

Week 15—SoulWise

When you are expecting a baby, you want to share your joy with the world. Naturally, you expect that everyone is going to be excited and supportive about your pregnancy. However, that is not always the case. Announcing your pregnant state can be disheartening to the woman who has struggled with infertility. Coworkers may resent the extra attention you're getting or any preferential treatment you may be receiving. A sibling might be jealous that you're having a baby before he or she does. Perhaps an older person is disapproving if they think you're having a child at too young or too old an age. As the old saying goes, "You're never going to please everybody." Be sensitive and considerate, but do not let others dampen your joy—and your celebration of the miracle of pregnancy and new life!

Am I disappointed in any specific person's reaction to my pregnancy? Why might the person have reacted as he or she did? How can I be more sensitive to that person's feelings?

_____

_____

_____

How has being pregnant affected my relationship with my family members? How do my parents feel about becoming grandparents? How do my siblings feel about being aunts and uncles?

_____

_____

_____

I know that I can't please everyone, and that some people may not be as happy for me as I'd like them to be. When this happens, I'll keep it from dampening my joy by doing the following:

_____

_____

_____

AMONG THIS WEEK'S WONDERS:

1:

Your baby practices sucking, swallowing, and breathing in preparation for her life outside the womb.

2:

Your baby's neck is now formed.

3:

Baby is making lots of motions now, from pursing her lips to clenching her fists, from curling her toes to turning her head.

THREE THINGS TO DO THIS WEEK:

1. *If a close friend or a family member is having a difficult time with my pregnancy, I'll make an effort to smooth things over with that person and restore our relationship.*

2. _____

3. _____

Week 16

Putting Baby First

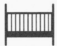

The sacrifices we make for our child during pregnancy are nature's way of preparing us for the job of parenting.

A **Word to the Mother-to-Be:** By week 16, your baby's limb movements are becoming more coordinated. Your baby now empties his bladder every forty to forty-five minutes. As the fetus continues its rapid development, you're sure to experience many signs that your body is hard at work too. One thing I discovered at this stage in my pregnancy was that there is an increased blood volume in the body to allow more oxygen to reach the fetus. I discovered this fact after feeling numbness in my hands and arms for several nights. Along the way in your pregnancy, you will experience new and sometimes uncomfortable sensations. Generally, you can rest assured that they are just a normal part of pregnancy. However, when an uncomfortable or unusual sensation lasts for more than a day or two, you should discuss it with your doctor. Chances are he or she will reassure you that there is nothing to worry about, but it's always best to check with your doctor if something feels a little out of the ordinary.

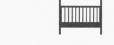

WEEK 16—BODYWISE

It seems that pregnancy affects nearly every part of a woman's body. I was shocked to find out that pregnancy even affected my sinuses. Suddenly, I was feeling congested all the time. Nasal congestion, sometimes accompanied by nosebleeds, is common for many women during pregnancy. These symptoms are caused by the increased blood flow to the mucous membranes of the nose (a result of pregnancy hormones). These problems are more common in the winter, when the air tends to be dry. Using a humidifier might relieve these nasal symptoms. If you get nosebleeds and they tend to be frequent or difficult to control, be sure to talk to your doctor. And if your nasal congestion becomes too uncomfortable to tolerate, discuss possible over-the-counter remedies with your doctor.

Have I experienced any new symptoms this week?

_____

_____

_____

Have I noticed any increased stuffiness? Has nasal congestion been keeping me from getting a good night's sleep?

_____

_____

Have I experienced any nosebleeds? How often do they occur? How do I get them to stop?

_____

_____

_____

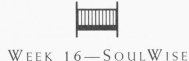

WEEK 16—SoulWise

You've been making sacrifices now for sixteen weeks (or at least since the week you found out you were pregnant). You've given up all drinks and foods that aren't good for a developing fetus, modified your exercise routine, and put away your 4-inch heels. Congratulations! You're learning that you can and will do everything it takes to protect and nurture your child. Parenting involves a multitude of sacrifices, and the things we give up during pregnancy are just nature's way of teaching us to put our child's well-being first—ahead of our own, if necessary. The experience of putting up with the little (or not so little) discomforts of pregnancy, the inconveniences, and the changes is a good way to prepare us for parenthood, when we'll often sacrifice our comfort for our child's. It also makes us grow in confidence that we're up to the task of parenting selflessly.

What sacrifices have I made during my pregnancy so far? Am I surprised at my willingness to make those sacrifices?

_____

_____

_____

What has been the most difficult change to make or discomfort to tolerate?

_____

_____

How confident am I in my ability and willingness to put my child's needs ahead of my own after he is born?

_____

_____

_____

Do I resent that my partner's sacrifices are minimal compared with mine right now? What kinds of sacrifices will he have to make once he becomes a father? Is he prepared to make them?

_____

_____

_____

AMONG THIS WEEK'S WONDERS:

1:

Baby's head and neck are becoming stronger and more aligned.

2:

While up until now baby's head was doing most of the growing, now the body is beginning to catch up.

3:

Your baby is now getting toenails.

4:

Baby is now almost 4 inches long.

THREE THINGS TO DO THIS WEEK:

1. Try to find a practical solution to a specific discomfort I'm experiencing, such as excessive nasal congestion.
2. Tell my partner why I think he'll be a great parent.
3. _____

Week 17

Making a Connection with My Baby

Feeling your baby move is sure to be one of the most memorable

experiences of your pregnancy. Be attentive

to these moments and cherish them.

A *Word to the Mother-to-Be*: During week 17, some moms-to-be begin feeling fetal movement. For me, the sensation happened one evening while I was reading my latest baby magazine. *Is that my baby moving or the taco I had for lunch?* I wondered.

My doctor had told me that I might begin to feel movement this week, so I was hoping this was it. Then, sure enough, it happened again. It was my baby moving! I was so excited by this new event, yet another milestone in my pregnancy. The movement was slight but unmistakable. This moment was sacred to me. From that point on, I paid more attention to the feel of things going on inside me. When I felt the little flutter, I tried to imagine what my baby was doing.

Feeling fetal movement is a great reminder to slow down and enjoy the experience of being pregnant. Try to tune in to everything that is happening inside you and focus on bonding with your baby. For me, my new awareness of my child inside me prompted me to start reading aloud, so that my baby could hear my voice and get to know it, and to be as aware of my presence as I was of hers.

WEEK 17—BODYWISE

Feeling your baby move inside you may be one of the most delightful experiences of your pregnancy. Although the embryo has been moving since week 7, most expectant mothers first become aware of the movement somewhere between weeks 18 and 22. So if you haven't yet felt movement, don't get impatient or feel anxious. Several factors can affect the detection of your baby's first movements. For example, a slender woman is likely to feel movements a little sooner than an overweight woman, and a woman who has had a baby before is likely to recognize movement earlier, because she knows what to expect.

Baby's early movements are usually far from dramatic and can be difficult to describe accurately. These movements might resemble a fluttering sensation or a rumbly tummy. The hard kicks to the ribs will come later. As you experience these subtle sensations more and more, you'll come to recognize them more readily.

If you've already experienced fetal movement, you know what a joyful experience it is. If you haven't yet, you can look forward to a milestone in your pregnancy that is sure to be one of the most memorable.

Have I noticed any sensations yet that might be fetal movement? What did they feel like?

_____

_____

_____

Have I been able to share any fetal movements with my partner? If so, what was his reaction?

_____

_____

_____

✎ *Have I sat in a quiet room with my hands on my belly to attempt to feel movement? What do I say to my baby to encourage her to move?*

_____

_____

_____

WEEK 17—SoulWise

If you tend to be a busy person, never sitting still for a moment, then your unborn baby can teach you to slow down. At this stage in your baby's development, if you want to feel her move, you need to be still and attentive. So put aside your to-do list for a while, find a quiet spot, and just sit with your hand on your belly. All of your concentration should be on your baby—not on the calls you need to make, the chores that need to be done, or the errands you need to run. All those things can wait; for now, just take a break to enjoy time with your child.

✎ *Do I have a tendency to always be busy? Is this a quality I like about myself, or would I prefer to learn to slow down? If so, how will I do this?*

_____

_____

_____

✎ *Am I learning to slow down and focus on my baby? What makes it hardest for me to do so?*

_____

_____

_____

✎ *How has being pregnant changed my perspective about what is really important in life?*

_____

_____

_____

✎ *What were my thoughts and feelings when I first felt my baby's movement inside me?*

_____

_____

_____

AMONG THIS WEEK'S WONDERS:

1:
Baby's growth really picks up speed in the next few weeks, although she still won't weigh more than half a pound.

2:
Baby's heart is pumping blood.

3:
The baby is developing reflexes, such as blinking, sucking, and swallowing.

4:
Your baby is the same size as her placenta. She'll outgrow it eventually, though.

THREE THINGS TO DO THIS WEEK:

1. *Take time to be still and be attentive to my baby.*
2. _____
3. _____

Week 18

Sharing the Bonds of Motherhood

To get the inside information on pregnancy, baby products,

and infant care, just talk to other moms.

A **Word to the Mother-to-Be:** The further along I got in my pregnancy, the more eager I was to learn about all the equipment I might need, from baby backpacks to interesting toys. I discovered that the best source of information on these issues was other moms. Mothers that I was meeting for the first time would eagerly offer up information, giving me straight answers to real questions. You ought to give this approach a try. You'd be surprised how willing other moms are to share what they know. As an example, I was very sure I was going to buy a certain brand of stroller—I'd even located the stores that sold them. So, I mentioned this purchase to a couple of moms with strollers I ran into while I shopped. Each came back with a similar suggestion: Buy a stroller that weighs less than 16 pounds because after the third time you've dug it out of your trunk, you'll wish you had! That was excellent advice. Try this approach to getting great pregnancy and baby product tips. Just ask any woman with a stroller how old her baby is just to break the ice. Then mention how far along you are and ask any baby-related questions, such as where she bought her stroller. Before you know it, you'll be getting information on baby formula, diapers, and maybe even breastfeeding advice.

WEEK 18—BODYWISE

During this time, as my baby was growing at a rapid pace, I was suddenly hungry all the time. Early on in my pregnancy, the sight and smell of food really turned me off. But now I rediscovered the joy of eating. Fresh fruit, crisp vegetables, pasta, steak— it all sounded good! A friend of mine, a mother of four, said she always knew she was pregnant when she craved butterscotch milkshakes. Many women have unusual cravings, although not all do. Just keep in mind that whether you're craving ice cream sundaes and hot dogs or pasta and vegetables, your increased appetite is not a reason to overeat or load up on junk food. Instead, you should eat high-nutrition foods that are good for your baby. Not only will high-calorie, low-nutrition foods be taking the place of the foods your baby really needs for his development, they'll also result in extra pounds that you'll be fighting to lose post-pregnancy.

Has my appetite increased lately? If I suffered from morning sickness, is it abating?

_____

_____

What are my most unusual cravings? Why do I suppose I crave these things?

_____

_____

_____

What are my favorite foods? What foods really turn me off? Have my food likes and dislikes changed dramatically?

_____

_____

_____

Week 18—SoulWise

Becoming a parent is bound to affect your relationship with your own mother, both positively and negatively. The mother–daughter relationship is complicated, no doubt about it. Even for those of us with a great mother–daughter relationship, our moms can often really push our buttons. If you feel your mother expresses her opinion a little too bluntly or has a tendency to meddle, the arrival of a grandchild may well bring out these characteristics even more. She'll naturally be eager to offer her advice and provide some guidance, but you might find that you're getting more of that than you want. It can take a delicate balancing act to include your mother in your new experience of motherhood while at the same time creating boundaries that are comfortable for both of you. But once you discover just how much you love your own child, you'll likely gain a new understanding and appreciation of what motivates your mom. In fact, your new perspective as a mom might even help you forge a new and richer relationship with your mother.

How would I characterize my relationship with my mother? Are we close, distant, back-and-forth?

_____

_____

_____

What about my mother-in-law, am I close to her? How can I make her be a part of my pregnancy?

_____

_____

_____

Do I plan to be a mother just like my own or will I parent my children differently? What changes will I make?

_____

_____

_____

AMONG THIS WEEK'S WONDERS:

1:
The pads of baby's fingers and toes begin to develop.

2:
Baby's bowel begins to receive early waste material (called *meconium*).

3:
Your baby now looks directly ahead instead of sideways.

4:
Your baby's bones are starting to harden.

5:
If you're having a boy, he now has a prostate gland.

6:
The nerves are being coated with myelin.

THREE THINGS TO DO THIS WEEK:

1. *Buy one indulgence food, but have just a small portion each day.*
2. *Do one thing to strengthen my relationship with my mother and show her how much she means to me.*
3. _____

Week 19

Getting Out and About

*This is a great time for you to schedule get-togethers
with family and friends.*

A Word to the Mother-to-Be: By week 19, your developing
baby has made some amazing progress. The fetus has now developed
reflexes, such as sucking and swallowing, and her body is becoming more in proportion with her head. If your baby is a girl, she now has egg cells in her ovaries. When I learned that all this was going on with my baby, I felt awed by the sheer wonder of Mother Nature and the miracle of carrying a little life within me. And because I was feeling great at this point in my pregnancy, I felt happier than ever. I was going out more, because I felt sick less, and was enjoying my pre-baby time to the fullest.

If you're in the "feeling great" stage of your pregnancy, as many women are in their second trimester, take advantage and *get out of the house!* As any mom with an infant can tell you, getting out of the house in those early weeks and months after your child is born will be tough. So make a point of getting out and enjoying yourself now. Plan romantic getaways with your partner, dinner with friends, shopping excursions, and anything else you feel like doing. Do these things now, before you get too big and uncomfortable, and before your newborn will demand all your time and attention.

WEEK 19—BODYWISE

As the fetus grows larger, you may start to experience back pain, usually centered in your lower back. This narrow part of your back is now balancing your enlarging uterus. Also at this point, your pelvic joints will begin to loosen in preparation for childbirth, and you might start feeling lower abdominal cramping as the ligaments supporting your uterus stretch. You can help minimize backache by maintaining good posture, elevating your legs when sitting, avoiding excess weight gain, and wearing comfortable low-heeled shoes. It's also important to avoid lifting with your back; bend at your knees instead. Also, make sure you're sleeping on a firm mattress that will support your back well. Consult your doctor if your back pain becomes unbearable. With back pain, abdominal pain, and achy pelvic joints, it is always helpful to get off your feet and sit or lie down in a comfortable position. Of course, tell your doctor if any of these discomforts become difficult to tolerate.

What is the most frequent pain I experience? What seems to instigate it?

_____

_____

_____

Did I have back problems before I got pregnant? Has my pregnancy made them flare up again? If so, have I consulted my doctor?

_____

_____

What have I found to be the best way to relieve my achy back, as well as other aches and pains? Do I take the necessary measures to be as comfortable as possible?

_____

_____

Week 19—SoulWise

This second trimester will most likely be the best part of your pregnancy. You are (hopefully) over your morning sickness and you feel less fatigued. You also haven't yet reached the uncomfortable aspects of the third trimester when the baby's large size causes more discomfort—and when you are outgrowing your maternity clothes. You also look pregnant now, so you're sure to get special treatment. Enjoy this time! Don't wish it away. Relish your growing shape, your shiny hair, and your glowing complexion. You'll want to revisit these lovely memories when you've just pulled an all-nighter trying to calm a restless baby.

How am I feeling emotionally during my second trimester?

_____

_____

_____

What are the best aspects of being nineteen weeks pregnant? What are the most difficult?

_____

_____

_____

Am I taking advantage of this "feeling good" time to enjoy my social life? What activities do I have planned for this week that will get me out of the house to enjoy pre-baby life?

_____

_____

_____

AMONG THIS WEEK'S WONDERS:

1:

Your baby's ears are now sticking out.

2:

Baby is now growing hair (called *lanugo*)—all over her body! Combined with a creamy substance called *vernix caseosa*, the hair protects your baby's skin.

3:

Your baby girl now has egg cells in her ovaries.

4:

Fingers and toes are well defined.

THREE THINGS TO DO THIS WEEK:

1. *Make plans for dinner with friends, a shopping excursion, or a romantic getaway with my partner (or all of these things).*
2. *Buy a good pair of comfortable shoes.*
3. _____

Week 20

Reaching the Halfway Mark

Baby's ears are fully developed, so go ahead and talk, read, and play music to him.

A *Word to the Mother-to-Be*: You've reached week 20. Congratulations! This means you are halfway through your pregnancy. By this week, your baby has started to practice breathing motions, even though his lungs are not developed enough to allow him to survive outside your body. His ears are fully functional and he enjoys all sorts of sounds, from abdominal noises to the sound of your voice. All your baby's organs are formed by now, and he is entering a period of simple growth. With your baby's increased size, by now you are likely to be feeling movement on a routine basis (although the excitement is anything but routine). You might even be able to tell whether your baby is awake or asleep based on his movements.

With the baby's growing size come new symptoms for his mother-to-be. Many expectant moms begin to experience shortness of breath at this time, caused by the uterus pressing into the lungs. Also around this time, it's not uncommon to begin waking up more than once at night because of the urge to urinate, again caused by the crowding of the internal organs—in this case the bladder—by the uterus.

Reaching the halfway mark in your pregnancy is exciting. It means that you've accomplished half your work of nurturing your unborn baby, and have gotten through half of the discomfort you'll experience. It also means that you're getting close to meeting your baby. This is definitely a milestone to celebrate.

Week 20 — BodyWise

Nobody ever said pregnancy was easy! Leg cramps, hemorrhoids, anemia, swelling, constipation, and gestational diabetes are some of the common complications of pregnancy. Fortunately, these side effects can often be controlled by certain modifications in your diet or lifestyle—such as avoiding excess weight gain, wearing comfortable shoes, and getting adequate rest and nutrition. The good news, of course, is that most, if not all, of the symptoms will vanish after you deliver. For now, do what you can to be as comfortable as possible, and keep your diet and lifestyle as healthy as possible to minimize the symptoms you may be experiencing. Most important, talk to your doctor if any discomfort you experience seems unusual or excessive.

Overall, how do I feel at this halfway point in my pregnancy?

_____

_____

_____

What unpleasant physical symptoms have I experienced with my pregnancy? What lifestyle or diet modifications have I made to control these side effects?

_____

_____

_____

Do I consistently follow a healthy nutritional plan? In what other ways am I working to ensure a healthy pregnancy?

_____

_____

WEEK 20—SoulWise

There is a lot of controversy about how much a baby understands in the womb. Some people believe playing classical music to their unborn child will increase his musical appreciation or give him a calmer temperament. Others are convinced that reading to their child while in the womb will improve his cognitive abilities. It's hard to know for sure how much of what is happening outside the womb affects your child; nevertheless, if you choose to try to stimulate your child's developing brain by reading to him or playing music, at the very least you will be developing a habit of focusing on ways to enrich your child and stimulate his intellectual development and curiosity about the world—a habit that will serve you and your child well in his growing years. So go ahead and get out your guitar or dig up your old poetry. After all, you do have a captive audience!

In what ways do I try to stimulate my baby's intellectual development?

_____

_____

_____

Have I noticed any response from my baby when I make extra efforts to communicate? Does he become more active when I play music or when he hears my voice?

_____

_____

_____

✏️ *Does my partner communicate with the baby? Does he do anything funny, like play the piano or turn the radio to a ball game, hoping our child will develop the talent or appreciate these things?*

_____

_____

_____

AMONG THIS WEEK'S WONDERS:

1:
Your baby is now getting eyebrows.

2:
Baby now has normal sleep cycles, just like a newborn. He will also settle into his favorite sleeping position.

3:
Your baby is starting to get hair on his head, although this may fall out several weeks after he is born.

4:
A baby girl now has a uterus.

5:
Baby now weighs about 10 ounces and is about 8 inches long.

THREE THINGS TO DO THIS WEEK:

1. *Select a favorite CD to play for my baby.*
2. *Make a list of unusual symptoms I'm experiencing and discuss them with my doctor.*
3. _____

Week 21

My Baby, the Action Hero!

*By this time, baby may be doing some amazing gymnastics—spinning,
turning, or somersaulting.*

A *Word to the Mother-to-Be:* By week 21, your baby is starting to test all of her new parts and is exploring her new capabilities. When she gets tired of all that activity, baby loves to fall asleep to the sound of your gastric juices churning or your voice singing.

At this stage of development, your baby has made amazing progress. At week 21, your baby can actually detect light. Doctors have confirmed that when an endoscope is inserted into the amniotic sac, a fetus will often try to protect her eyes from the light on the instrument, either by turning away or by using her hands and fingers to shield her face. Your little one can detect when you are in a well-lighted place versus a dark room.

Your baby has also discovered other things that she prefers. For example, by week 21, she already has a preference for her favorite position. Your baby will decide whether she wants to sleep with her little chin resting on her chest or with her head back. She will even decide if she likes to fall asleep with a hand to her face, or while sucking a finger. By the way, thumb sucking is a routine event at this stage, preparing your baby for the important work of nursing when she is born.

Your baby may also be doing some amazing gymnastics—spinning, turning, or somersaulting. If you haven't felt powerful jabs and kicks yet, you'll be feeling them all the time before too long.

WEEK 21—BodyWise

By this time in your pregnancy, getting a good night's sleep is likely to be a challenge. Your sleep position can affect not only how well you sleep but also how well you feel overall. If you're in the habit of sleeping on your back, it's time for a change. Sleeping on your back means that the entire weight of your uterus is resting on your back, intestines, and the inferior vena cava, which can hamper circulation. This can result in back pain, hemorrhoids, breathing and circulation difficulties, and even cause low blood pressure. A great position to sleep in is lying on your left side, preferably with one leg crossed over the other and a pillow between your legs. That way, you can maximize blood flow to the baby and improve kidney function and the collection and elimination of waste, thereby reducing any swelling in your legs and feet.

✎ *What position have I been sleeping in? Have I tried sleeping on my left side with a pillow between my legs? Has that made my sleep more restful?*

_____

_____

_____

✎ *Do I have any swelling in my ankles or feet? Have I mentioned this swelling to my doctor?*

_____

_____

✎ *What do I like best about my pregnant body?*

_____

_____

_____

WEEK 21—SoulWise

A close and loving extended family can be a real blessing in a child's life. Whether aunts and uncles, grandparents, cousins, or even godparents, time spent with these people can be special and joyful for your child, and their affection can enhance her sense of confidence and trust in the world around her. If you and your partner have good relationships with your families, you can look forward to bringing your child into the warm, loving environment that you share with them. If you're estranged from certain family members, consider whether you want your child to experience the tension that situation may cause, or if you want her to be deprived of a relationship with these people. Now would be a good time to mend fences and start anew if you feel it is appropriate to do so. Your pregnancy may be the perfect icebreaker. Consider sharing news of the event as a way to initiate contact and overcome any discord that exists between you and members of your or your partner's family.

In what ways can I use this special time of pregnancy to draw closer to each of my baby's grandparents? Have I made them feel a part of this important event in my life by sharing my plans, concerns, and excitement with them?

_____

_____

_____

Is there anyone who either because of distance or conflict may not be as involved in my child's life as I would like? How can I change this situation?

_____

_____

_____

Who in our extended family do I expect to be an important part of my child's life and a good influence on her?

_____

_____

AMONG THIS WEEK'S WONDERS:

1:
The baby can now control her movements in the amniotic fluid.
She may be spinning, turning, or doing somersaults.

2:
Your baby's heartbeat is now so strong that it can be heard
with a common stethoscope.

3:
Your baby's legs will reach their final proportions.

4:
Your baby is getting hairier as lanugo spreads all over her body.

5:
Baby sucks her thumb in preparation for nursing once outside the womb.

THREE THINGS TO DO THIS WEEK:

1. Work on mending fences with a family member with whom I am having difficulties but want to have in my child's life.
2. Make a point of sharing some baby plans with the grandparents-to-be.
3. _____

Week 22

Getting a Good Education

Now may be the time to add baby and parenting

magazine subscriptons.

A *Word to the Mother-to-Be*: There is so much for a first-time mom to learn. From how to deal with diaper rash to how frequently a baby needs to nurse to how to get a fussy baby to sleep, I was a true beginner. Whenever I went to see my obstetrician, I found myself poring over all the magazines for expectant mothers and parents of young children that I could get my hands on. After finding that I didn't have enough time to do all my reading while I waited to see the doctor, I decided to subscribe to a few magazines of my own.

Soon a variety of magazines arrived. I loved the day my first baby magazine came in the mail. It was a different feeling for me, getting rid of my stack of women's fashion magazines and seeing a stack of baby magazines take their place. But this was a change I was willing to make. I knew these magazines would be useful—make that necessary—to educate me about all the child-care issues I was beginning to be curious about.

How about you? What reading material are you finding most useful as you look ahead to motherhood? Whether in magazines, books, or newspaper articles by child-care experts, there are abundant sources of information to help new moms. You will be surprised how many helpful tips you can pick up, so that when you encounter new situations with your baby, you'll feel more knowledgeable and confident. Also realize that you have valuable insight of your own when it comes to your child, and learn to trust your own judgment.

WEEK 22—BODYWISE

When I was pregnant, I was always hot. No, I don't mean sexy (although pregnant women can be that, too), but I literally always felt warm. My baby was quite the little heater. Women who are in late pregnancy during the hot summer months may find themselves especially uncomfortable. There is not much you can do except what you've always done to stay cool, which is to wear loose, light clothing; enjoy a cool shower or swim; stay in the air conditioning; and invest in a good fan!

Do I feel like I'm always warm? Does this make me irritable? What should I do to keep the heat from making me cranky?

_____

_____

_____

What do I like about being pregnant during this time of year? What do I dislike?

_____

_____

_____

Am I having trouble sleeping because I get warm at night? What have I done to deal with this situation? Has this affected my sleeping arrangements with my partner?

_____

_____

_____

WEEK 22—SOULWISE

Now that you and your partner have adjusted to the news that you're going to be parents, how are things going between the two of you? Relationships naturally go through highs and lows, but major life-changing events, such as expecting (and having) a baby, can be particularly significant. Your partner and you might be on cloud nine right now as you both eagerly anticipate the bundle of joy that you've created. Or perhaps he is stressed out about how you're going to meet all the financial obligations that come with raising a child. Financial difficulty can make pregnancy a particularly stressful time. But no matter what the situation is between you and your partner, communication is key. Encourage him to share his worries, and do all that you can to get him to focus on the joy of the new addition to your family. It's important to work out any conflicts or concerns before your baby is born so that you can bring him into a loving, harmonious home, free of anger and discord.

How is my partner feeling about impending parenthood now? Have his feelings changed since he first found out? Is he more excited? More stressed?

_____

_____

_____

Are there issues I'd like to resolve with my partner, such as getting him to stop smoking or to spend less time at work? Can I convince him that healthy habits will be good for our family?

_____

_____

_____

Realistically, do I think that having a baby will strengthen our relationship or present new challenges for us to overcome?

_____

_____

_____

AMONG THIS WEEK'S WONDERS:

1:

Baby can hear your digestive system and the swishing from your major blood vessels, and he can also hear sounds from outside the womb, such as music playing and the voices of other people.

2:

Your baby is trying to blink even though his eyes can't open yet.

3:

Baby's skeleton is turning into bone.

4:

Your baby weighs about 15 ounces and is about 10 inches long.

5:

Your baby's brain is growing very quickly now.

THREE THINGS TO DO THIS WEEK:

1. *Buy a pregnancy swimsuit if summer is approaching.*
2. *Subscribe to magazines for expectant and new mothers.*
3. _____

Week 23

Looking Forward to Baby, but Enjoying Pre-Baby Time

As you can imagine, traveling with an infant is just not as carefree

as it is pre-baby. So why not plan a getaway now?

A *Word to the Mother-to-Be:* No doubt you've begun to make preliminary plans for your baby's birth, coming up with ideas for the nursery, considering decisions about whether to return to work or be a stay-at-home mom, and thinking about child-care arrangements if you will be working outside of your home. As you make plans for your baby's birth and beyond, think too about things that you would like to do before the baby's birth. One activity you'll definitely be less free to participate in after the baby's birth is travel. As you can imagine, travel with an infant and her accoutrements is just not as carefree as it was pre-baby. So why not plan a trip for yourself and your partner and get away for a long weekend or even a week-long trip. At this point, you're not yet feeling as encumbered as you will be in your third trimester, especially the last month or two, and you're probably feeling pretty good overall. So take advantage of it. There are, of course, certain precautions you should take. For example, don't travel to a very hot location, as that will probably be uncomfortable; avoid destinations at a high altitude, as the reduced oxygen may be a difficulty for you and the baby; and avoid travel that would require vaccination. In other words, as long as you don't plan any extreme travel, a getaway can be the perfect treat. Just be sure to let your doctor know of your plans and get his or her okay.

WEEK 23—BODY WISE

Let's talk about sex! Chances are that you've had some questions about it during your pregnancy. Is sex allowed? Will sex hurt the baby? Is it okay to have an orgasm? With your growing belly, you and your partner may need to be more creative at finding comfortable positions. For most women, sex during pregnancy is fine, but be sure to okay it with your doctor. Sometimes, if a woman has certain conditions, is considered a high-risk pregnancy, or is expecting multiples, her physician may advise against sexual relations. Immediately report any bleeding or pain you may experience. If your doctor gives the green light, enjoy your sex life while you can. Chances are, after the baby is born, your fatigue may slow you down for a while, and when your head hits the pillow, the last thing you'll be thinking about is sex.

Do I have any fears about having sex now that I'm pregnant? Am I afraid the baby will get hurt, or am I more cautious about being too active?

_____

_____

What about my partner? Is he afraid he'll hurt the baby? Is he less—or more—attracted to me now that I'm pregnant?

_____

_____

Have I had any problems during sex, such as increased pain or any bleeding, that I should report to my doctor?

_____

_____

_____

WEEK 23—SoulWise

Without a doubt, your baby is never far from your thoughts right now. It may sometimes seem that the world revolves around your baby—before she is even born.
Being focused on your unborn child is obviously a healthy and important response
to be being pregnant. When your baby is born, she will become the center of your
universe even more. So while you can, take advantage of your pre-baby time to do
something special for yourself. Whether you choose to take a romantic trip with
your partner, travel to see a friend you haven't seen in a while, or get away for a
"girlfriends' weekend," take a break to spend some time just the way you want to
spend it.

*What would be my ideal way to spend a long weekend away right now? With whom
would I want to spend it and where?*

_____

_____

_____

Do I feel up to taking a trip? What are my concerns about travel right now?

_____

_____

_____

What do I expect to be the most dramatic changes in my life when my baby is born?

_____

_____

_____

Have my partner and I been making plans for romantic time together? Do we spend enough quality time together?

_____

_____

_____

THREE THINGS TO DO THIS WEEK:

1. *Plan a special trip for me and my partner.*
2. *Seduce my partner tonight!*
3. _____

Week 24

Getting Ready for Baby

Now is a good time to get rid of physical and emotional clutter.

A **Word to the Mother-to-Be:** Now that you've reached week 24 of your pregnancy, there's a good chance you've already experienced the "nesting" impulse. Although some women don't experience this impulse until late in their pregnancies, by week 24 I was definitely in nesting mode. Much like the name suggests, nesting is an urge to prepare a comfy, cozy place for your child. It's really all about housekeeping. For many pregnant women, they catch up on all the cleaning they've been meaning to do for months, if not years, during this time. It's the time to organize drawers and shelves, clean out closets, and discard old belongings that are no longer useful. For me, nesting was all about going through all my closets to reorganize and get rid of clutter. I packed up bag after bag of things I just didn't need anymore and donated them to a local charity. It felt great to have my house in order as I prepared for the newest member of the family.

If you haven't yet had the urge to go through every closet, shelf, and drawer in your home and reorganize it, chances are you will soon. In addition, nesting will probably entail lots of fussing over the nursery—thinking about colors and patterns, or maybe even looking at paint and fabric swatches. Whatever activities nesting entails for you, it's sure to be just one more way for you to feel even more connected to the idea that soon you'll be bringing your baby home.

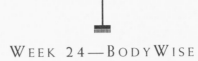

Week 24—BodyWise

Between weeks 24 and 28, your doctor may order a glucose tolerance test to determine if you have gestational diabetes. About 2 percent of pregnant women develop this condition. It is one of the most common complications of pregnancy. Those at higher risk for this condition include older pregnant women, women with a family history of diabetes, and women who are obese. Moms-to-be who develop gestational diabetes can have normal pregnancies and healthy babies when their blood sugar is closely controlled through diet and, if needed, medication. Blood sugar abnormalities disappear after delivery in all but 2 or 3 percent of women.

Am I in a high-risk group for gestational diabetes? Have I been tested for the condition yet?

_____

_____

_____

What general health concerns related to my pregnancy do I have that I should discuss with my doctor?

_____

_____

_____

Do I know what choices I have when it comes to my delivery? If not, how can I become better informed?

_____

_____

_____

WEEK 24—SoulWise

As you go through your home to organize and eliminate clutter, think too about emotional clutter with which you may need to deal. If you're facing any conflicts with family members or your partner that are causing you stress during what should be a time of happiness in your life, decide what you should do about it—and then do it. Perhaps you'll decide to just accept the situation and move on. Or you might choose to speak to the person with whom you're having a conflict and come to a mutually acceptable resolution. The important thing is to choose a course of action that will truly give you peace of mind by eliminating the anxiety or stress that the situation may be causing for you. This will make it easier for you to focus on the excitement of having a baby. In addition, you might also develop a better relationship with someone with whom you haven't been seeing eye to eye.

Is there anyone with whom I am having a difficult relationship at this time? What is the cause of this conflict?

_____

_____

What is the best course of action for handling this situation? Am I prepared to follow through on it?

_____

_____

What would be the benefits of amending this situation? Do I believe this will be a lasting resolution?

_____

_____

_____

1:

Baby gains over 6 ounces this week and could top 1 pound 5 ounces by week's end.

2:

Your baby's wrinkly skin starts smoothing out as more fat forms.
Baby's thin skin is still transparent.

3:

Baby's brain begins rapid growth.

4:

Your baby has taste buds on his tongue and even inside his cheeks.

5:

Baby's breastbone becomes "bony."

THREE THINGS TO DO THIS WEEK:

1. *Determine a course of action for dealing with a difficult relationship, and follow through on it.*
2. *Continue to follow a sensible eating plan.*
3. _____

Week 25

Thinking About Labor

It's natural to worry about labor, but don't spend too much time worrying about it. Instead, make preparations for labor and delivery by attending childbirth classes and keeping fit.

A *Word to the Mother-to-Be:* You are now well into your sixth month of pregnancy, approaching the end of your second trimester. This may be a good time to talk about childbirth. No doubt you've begun to think about this subject—with excitement, of course, but probably also with some anxiety about the pain and how you'll handle it. It is natural to worry about (and even dread) labor. Of course, though, worrying about labor too much is not particularly helpful. The best way to deal with this part of having a baby is to be as relaxed about it as possible. This doesn't mean you should be in denial and avoid thinking about it until you're actually in labor. Instead, it means you should be realistic about the fact that labor can be very painful, but also that you should focus on what you can do to make it more bearable. For instance, you can decide now who will be your labor coach (if not your partner, choose a close friend who won't be overwhelmed) and attend childbirth classes together. Also, you can realistically think about painkillers as an option to relieve or lessen labor pain. It is comforting to know that you can accept pain relief if you want it when the time comes.

Another way to take a proactive role in making your labor easier is to stay fit. It isn't necessary to hire a personal trainer to guide you through a daily workout, but you should follow a suitable pregnancy workout routine. (Talk to your doctor about an exercise program if you haven't already done so.) If walking is more your thing than a workout, make an effort to take a daily walk.

WEEK 25 — BODY WISE

Being pregnant can make you tired, but now is not the time to neglect your exercise. Assuming the doctor says it's okay, make sure you get out and about. Walking is great for staying in shape while you're pregnant, and, as mentioned earlier, a great way to keep fit for labor. You can fit walking into your everyday schedule. For example, when you go to the store, ignore those tempting parking spots near the door and park in the back of the lot. The walk will do you good! When your partner gets home, ask him to take a walk with you. (If the weather is poor, head to the mall for a stroll.) Exercising will help you to be more fit to deliver your baby, and it will also increase your stamina once the baby is born.

How am I feeling this week? Do I feel up to following an exercise routine? If not, could this be because I haven't been active enough so far in my pregnancy?

_____

_____

_____

What am I doing to stay fit during my pregnancy? Should I be doing more?

_____

_____

Whom can I ask to be my exercise buddy? Have I considered joining a fitness group for expectant moms?

_____

_____

WEEK 25—SOULWISE

Now that you're this far along in your pregnancy, you probably find yourself wondering what you'll be like as a mom. This is especially likely to be the case if you're having your first child. Some women approach their impending motherhood with a great deal of confidence, others with some anxiety. If you're among the latter, my first piece of advice to you is "Relax!" Have confidence in yourself and in your instincts as a parent. You may not have all the answers now, but when you're caring for your child, chances are you'll know what to do. And in those instances when you just can't figure it out on your own, there are plenty of people who will be willing to help, such as your baby's grandmothers, your sisters or girlfriends who've already had babies, and your pediatrician. Know that you don't have to be supermom and have all the answers all the time.

Do I worry that I won't know the "right" way to care for my baby? Do I feel inexperienced or do I lack confidence about my mothering abilities? How can I overcome these feelings?

_____

_____

Do I believe in maternal instinct? If so, do I feel I'll have it when I become a mother?

_____

_____

Will I be willing to ask for help when I just don't know how to handle a specific situation with my baby? Who am I most likely to turn to?

_____

_____

_____

✎ *Who is my role model for being a good mother? Which of her qualities as a mother do I most admire?*

_____

_____

AMONG THIS WEEK'S WONDERS:

1:
Baby weighs about 1 pound 9 ounces.

2:
Your baby is establishing a strong grip.

3:
Baby's nails—both on fingers and toes—continue to grow.

4:
Baby's capillaries are forming, and blood vessels develop in the lungs.

5:
The baby's nostrils are opening.

6:
Baby is getting buds for her permanent (not baby!) teeth.

THREE THINGS TO DO THIS WEEK:

1. *Choose a pregnancy exercise plan and follow it.*
2. *Share concerns that I have about caring for an infant with my mother, sister, or a girlfriend, and solicit some advice.*
3. _____

Week 26

Developing a Birth Plan

You have more choices than you realize when it comes to childbirth.

Being informed about your options will allow you

to make choices that are right for you.

A *Word to the Mother-to-Be:* Now that we've talked about labor and the importance of the physical and mental readiness for it, let's take the delivery talk one step further. When I was in my sixth month of pregnancy and looking very pregnant, other moms-to-be began to ask me how I was going to give birth. Well, up to this point, I hadn't really thought about it. "What's your birth plan?" they would ask. "Are you going to have a vaginal birth or a C-section?" "Have you selected the music you want played in the delivery room?" "Who's going to cut the umbilical cord?" and "Are you taking a doula into the delivery room with you?" And so on. All these questions made me realize that my husband and I had some planning to do and some decisions to make.

Yes, it was time to do my homework. By speaking to my doctor and reading pregnancy guides, I began learning about all my options and what decisions I needed to make. I made a list, and then researched the pros and cons of each choice. My husband and I then discussed each issue and made our decisions. As you can imagine, there is a lot to think about when it comes to giving birth. Take time to learn what questions you need to ask so that you get the answers you need. Then consider your options carefully and choose the ones that are best suited for you and with which you will be the most comfortable.

WEEK 26—BODYWISE

By week 26 of your pregnancy, you are likely to be gaining weight more steadily. You may be gaining at a rate of a pound a week from this point on. The extra weight could start to take its toll on your back. Some things you can do to reduce back pain include wearing low-healed shoes, avoiding sitting or standing for extended periods of time, and using a footstool to raise your knees higher than your hips when you sit. And since you're in a period of quicker weight gain, now may be a good time to think about how well you've done so far with sticking to a high-nutrition diet that is low on empty calories. Renew your commitment to eating well for yourself and your baby.

Have I been experiencing back pain? Has this become more of an issue for me at this point in my pregnancy? What am I doing about it?

_____

_____

_____

Am I continuing to follow a sound nutrition plan? Is it easy, or am I getting tired of it?

_____

_____

Have I discovered any new recipes since I've started watching my eating more carefully? Which ones are my favorites?

_____

_____

_____

WEEK 26—SoulWise

It is important to nurture your relationship with your partner during this time. Even though you're creating a family, you're still a couple, too! It is important to maintain the intimacy you share. Start developing good habits now that will help keep your relationship strong even during your baby's infancy, when time alone with your partner will be a precious commodity. Set aside time each day to just spend time together, whether it is to take a walk, enjoy a meal and conversation, or engage in a hobby together. Make a point of doing thoughtful things to make your partner feel special. For example, put a loving note in his briefcase or lunch bag, prepare a candlelit dinner for an evening after work, or surprise him with a thoughtful gift. Make sure he knows how important he is to you and that you won't be forgetting about him, even when a newborn will be demanding so much of your attention.

Am I giving my partner and our relationship the attention I should be? What should I be doing differently? In what ways has my being pregnant increased our love and commitment to one another?

_____

_____

_____

What activities can my partner and I share that will draw us closer together? What can we do to maintain the closeness even during the early months of caring for a newborn?

_____

_____

_____

Am I concerned about the health of our relationship once the baby is born? Will we have to work harder to maintain "couple time"?

_____

_____

_____

AMONG THIS WEEK'S WONDERS:

1:
Your baby is practicing his breathing.

2:
Air sacs are developing in baby's lungs, which are now secreting surfactant to keep the tissues from sticking together.

3:
Baby is developing more brain wave activity, especially in his auditory and visual systems.

4:
You can now see baby's fingernails.

5:
Baby's hair follicles begin to form this month.

THREE THINGS TO DO THIS WEEK:

1. *Make a list of the birthing decisions I need to make and start researching my options so I can make informed decisions.*
2. *Plan a romantic evening with my partner.*
3. _____

W e e k 2 7

Working with a Doula

Meeting with a doula helped me move beyond my fears and

get back in tune with the joys of expectant motherhood.

A *Word to the Mother-to-Be:* Of all the options I had with regard to my child's birth, I was most intrigued by the idea of having a doula assist me during childbirth. In doing some research, I discovered that a doula is a professionally trained person who assists expectant parents in thinking through and creating their birth plan. And if the expectant parents wish, the doula can stay by the side of the laboring mom throughout her entire labor. In the delivery room, the doula's role is to provide emotional support, physical comfort in whatever ways she is able, and an objective viewpoint in communications with the medical staff. I felt that having a doula might enhance my childbirth experience and began my search for one with whom I could work.

When I first met with my doula, I had a long list of questions for her. Tracy also took time to ask me questions that helped her build a framework for our relationship. We talked about the pros and cons of many approaches and choices. She provided me with her cell phone number and said to call day or night for any reason or concern. She guaranteed me that the moment I was in labor, she would either come to my house or meet me at the hospital, depending on what I wanted. She would never leave my side, and would stay with me until the baby and I were safely and comfortably in our recovery room. She would even stay to assist in the first breastfeeding if I needed her help.

A doula is not the right choice for every woman, but for me the idea of having a pregnancy and delivery guide was very appealing. Perhaps this option intrigues you, too. If so, take time to learn more about doulas. If you choose to work with a doula, be sure to find one with whom you feel comfortable and one who will provide the kind of support and reassurance you need.

WEEK 27—BODYWISE

One of the issues I discussed with my doula was breastfeeding versus bottle-feeding. As most women probably know by now, breast milk is nature's perfect food for small babies. There is a long list of reasons why breast milk is better than formula. Some key reasons are that breast milk has ingredients that cannot be duplicated in commercial formulas and is more easily digested by infants. Nursed babies are less likely to have digestive difficulties such as constipation or diarrhea. Also, on a practical note, when you're waking up for 2 A.M. feedings, it's a lot easier to breastfeed than to go to the kitchen and warm up a bottle—all while the baby is crying. Of course, the choice between breastfeeding and bottle-feeding is a personal one. Learn more about the pros and cons of each method and make the decision that suits your and your baby's needs.

Have I decided to breastfeed or use a bottle? What are my reasons for this decision?

_____

_____

_____

How will I feel if I try breastfeeding but am not successful due to a lack of milk or other reasons? Will I be disappointed that I have to switch to a bottle or proud that I at least gave it a try?

_____

_____

✏️ *If I have elected to breastfeed, how long do I anticipate I'll be doing so? If I'm returning to work, do I plan to continue breastfeeding then?*

_____

_____

WEEK 27—SOULWISE

As you consider all your options regarding childbirth and child care, you may start to feel a little overwhelmed or even a little insecure about whether you're making the best decisions. If that happens, allow yourself a break from decision making. You don't have to know everything now, and you certainly don't have to figure it all out on your own. Become well informed by reading pregnancy and infant-care guides and by talking to experienced moms you trust. Most of all, trust yourself to make choices that will be best for you and your baby. Chances are some of the decisions you fret about in advance will seem like no-brainers by the time you actually have to make them.

✏️ *Do I feel insecure that I will make the wrong choices about my birth options? Why?*

_____

_____

_____

✏️ *Have I spoken to other women about their choices and why they made these decisions? Did this help me to understand my options more clearly?*

_____

_____

_____

How will I feel if any of my choices don't work out? If I ask for an epidural after initially refusing one, will I feel like a failure or accept this as the right choice for me?

_____

_____

_____

AMONG THIS WEEK'S WONDERS:

1:
Baby's brain continues its rapid development.

2:
Your baby will grow half an inch this week.

3:
Eyelids begin to open and the retina begins to form.

4:
The lungs and brain continue their development.

5:
As baby grows stronger, you'll be feeling much more vigorous kicks.

THREE THINGS TO DO THIS WEEK:

1. Gather and read information about breastfeeding and bottle-feeding.
2. Consult with my partner about our birth plans and put them in writing. Be prepared to discuss our options with my doctor.
3. _____

Week 28

I'm Well on My Way

Now may be the time to allow siblings to bond with the new baby
by feeling his kicks and jabs.

A Word to the Mother-to-Be: Welcome to the third trimester! By now, your baby is about 13 inches long and weighs close to 2 pounds. His movements are probably easy to detect, especially when you're in a relaxed position. This is partly because when you're busy and on the move, your baby is lulled by the motion and your own attention is focused elsewhere. (By the ninth month, the bigger knees and elbows and the stronger movements will be hard to miss no matter what you're doing.) When you settle down, your baby may suddenly become more active. Your baby's movements are dependent on you in other ways as well. For example, baby's activity may increase after you have a snack, particularly if you have a sweet snack. You might also notice that your baby is more active if you are anxious or excited, in response to the increased adrenaline. Although weeks 24 to 28 tend to be a fetus's most active, movement still tends to be erratic. Nevertheless, at this point you should expect to feel your baby's movement at various times throughout the day.

By week 28, it will probably become possible for others to feel the baby's movements by putting a hand on your tummy. Just as it's thrilling for you the first time you feel your baby kick, it is also exciting for other family members to experience the baby's movements. Now may be the time to allow siblings to bond with the new baby by feeling his kicks and jabs.

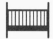

WEEK 28 — BODYWISE

Between weeks 28 and 36, your doctor will probably be seeing you every two weeks. (After week 36, you'll be seeing your doctor on a weekly basis.) Your doctor will be checking the size and height of your uterus and whether you've begun to dilate, taking your blood pressure, examining any swelling, and checking very closely for any signs of labor or fetal distress. (All this extra attention really makes it sink in that the baby will be here very soon!)

How am I feeling? What questions do I have for the doctor for my next visit?

_____

_____

What things did my doctor check for on my last visit? Did he or she monitor anything that hadn't been checked before?

_____

_____

Has my partner been attending my doctor's visits with me? How does he feel about being in the home stretch of the pregnancy?

_____

_____

_____

Does the doctor have any concerns that he or she wishes to monitor more closely? What specific advice did my doctor give me on my last visit?

_____

_____

WEEK 28—SoulWise

I discovered another unusual side effect of being pregnant: strange and frequent dreams. Suddenly, I was having all kinds of dreams that made very little sense. My friends tell me the same thing happened to them. One of my pregnant friends dreamed she gave birth to a litter of puppies! Another dreamed that she forgot her baby at the zoo, and a mother elephant took him in. These dreams can be quite humorous, yet disturbing, too. Experts say they are a reflection of our increasing worries about our child. For instance, dreams of having puppies or other animals may reflect a concern that your child will have something wrong with him. Dreams that something happened to the baby are common because we worry that we will fail to keep the baby safe. Strange dreams during pregnancy are a natural expression of the anxiety we feel.

What is the strangest dream I've had during pregnancy? What do I think it means?

_____

_____

_____

_____

_____

Do I sometimes worry about my baby's health or welfare, or about the great responsibility of being a mother? Do I see a connection between these worries and my dreams? Do I remember to call upon my faith to give me peace of mind?

_____

_____

_____

_____

✎ *Have I compared dream stories with my girlfriends? What are some of the most unusual or funny ones I've heard?*

_____

_____

_____

AMONG THIS WEEK'S WONDERS:

1:
Baby is developing stronger muscle tone, including a good grip!

2:
The baby's eyelids are opening and no longer fused together. Any day now, the eyes will be completely developed.

3:
Your baby's lungs can now breathe air—a good thing to know in case he arrives early.

4:
Your baby's movements may be waking you up now.

5:
Baby is almost 13 inches long and weighs about 2 pounds.

THREE THINGS TO DO THIS WEEK:

1. *Spend more time off my feet, and elevate my legs when I'm sitting.*
2. *Keep a pad of paper by my bed so I can record my dreams and try to analyze what they mean.*
3. _____

Week 29

Growing a Little Impatient

Along with the excitement and joy of being pregnant, it is also not unusual to feel weary and eager for the pregnancy to be over with.

A *Word to the Mother-to-Be:* I'm sure I don't need to tell you that you've accomplished a lot in the past six and a half months. By now, your baby has achieved enough development so that if born early, she has a real chance of survival. But, of course, there's more work to be done.

As your baby continues to grow, the demands on your body will continue to increase. In addition to symptoms you've already been experiencing—such as mild swelling of your hands and feet, shortness of breath, and difficulty sleeping (which may now be intensified)—you may also begin to experience new symptoms, such as varicose veins in your legs and lower abdominal aches.

By now, you may also be feeling weary or even bored with the pregnancy and eager for it to reach its fruitful end. This is a natural feeling in the later stages of pregnancy, and may occur even more frequently as you near your due date. When you start to feel this way, realize that it is another perfectly normal emotion that accompanies pregnancy. One good way to deal with this feeling is to allow yourself time to focus on something else. Find an activity you enjoy that has nothing to do with either being pregnant or preparing for a newborn. For example, instead of shopping for baby equipment, shop for something for yourself or for your home— even if you have to shop online to avoid spending too much time on your feet.

WEEK 29—BODYWISE

Another symptom that may develop in the last trimester of pregnancy is sciatica. The pressure of the growing fetus and enlarged uterus can also affect the sciatic nerve, resulting in lower back, buttocks, and leg pain. If you experience sciatica, the best way to deal with it is to avoid being on your feet for prolonged periods of time. You might also apply moist heat to your lower back for pain relief. Sciatic pain during pregnancy is not always persistent; instead, it may come and go depending on the position of the baby. It might last for a period of several days at a time and vanish for extended periods of time as well. If you experience sciatic pain, be sure to discuss it with your doctor, especially if you experience prolonged or intense pain.

Overall, how am I feeling? What new symptoms am I experiencing most frequently?

_____

_____

_____

Have I been experiencing sciatica? What am I doing to relieve it?

_____

_____

_____

How much weight have I gained so far? Is my weight gain within the proper range? Am I eating well enough to nourish my growing child?

_____

_____

_____

Am I getting sufficient rest, or am I pushing myself to do too much? Do I listen to my body's signals to get more rest?

_____

_____

WEEK 29—SOULWISE

One of the factors that may contribute to a sense of weariness or boredom with pregnancy is a tendency for the state of pregnancy to become a characteristic that defines the pregnant woman. Sometimes, it may seem as if your pregnancy is all other people can talk to you about. If you start to feel frustrated by this trend, take proactive steps to let people know that you do actually still have other interests. You might politely suggest a change of topic or redirect the conversation to something in which you and the other person or persons share an interest. The converse situation is, of course, a pregnant woman who expects other people to be as passionate about her pregnancy as she is. If you catch yourself chattering away about your pregnancy at every opportunity, be sensitive to the fact that while your pregnancy is one of the most important events in your life, it doesn't have the same significance for most other people you know or encounter.

Am I impatient for my pregnancy to be over with? When do I feel the most impatient?

_____

_____

Do other people seem to think of me as being "the pregnant woman" rather than thinking of all my other qualities and interests? How do I redirect their questions and conversations?

_____

_____

What is my favorite non-pregnancy-related way to spend time? Do I make enough time for this activity and other activities that interest me?

_____

_____

_____

AMONG THIS WEEK'S WONDERS:

1:
Baby's brain is now capable of directing breathing and controlling her body temperature.

2:
Baby's skin will smooth out as more fat is deposited beneath the surface.

3:
Your baby's senses of taste, smell, hearing, and seeing are becoming better.

4:
Your baby has eyelashes!

THREE THINGS TO DO THIS WEEK:

1. *Make plans for an activity that has nothing to do with pregnancy or baby care.*
2. _____
3. _____

Week 30

Learning to Be a (Great!) Parent

How would you describe the qualities of a good parent?

A *Word to the Mother-to-Be:* During my pregnancy, I was really diligent about providing for my baby the best possible inside environment I could. I took good care of my health and made it a point to stay positive and in a good frame of mind. I kept all my doctor's appointments and closely followed recommendations for ensuring the best possible pregnancy. My goal was to do my part in all possible ways to have a healthy baby—and one, I hoped, with a good disposition! I also thought a lot about parenting my little girl and being the best parent I could be.

A great way to think about how you'll parent your child in a way that will ensure raising a happy, secure, and well-adjusted child is to observe parents whose child-rearing style you admire. You may also think about specific parenting techniques your mom used that you want to emulate. You can also increase your parenting know-how and confidence by reading a parenting guide you trust. The point is that the more you know, the more secure you'll feel. So educate yourself and you'll have less reason to feel insecure. Most of all, though, learn to trust your instincts. Trust yourself to know how to handle specific parenting issues as they arise. Also know that you don't have to have all the answers. Allow yourself to turn to others for guidance whenever you need it.

WEEK 30—BODYWISE

Have you had any swelling in your hands or feet yet? As you get further into the third trimester and your baby puts more pressure on your body, the chances for swelling become greater. Many women find they must remove their wedding ring because it has become too tight. You may also find that even your once-comfortable shoes don't fit as comfortably anymore. Most of the time, the swelling is completely normal and not a cause for concern, but have your doctor monitor it to make sure you're okay. You can help keep the swelling down by staying off your feet, elevating your legs, and cutting back on your salt intake. Some women are lucky and experience little or no swelling during pregnancy, or experience it only as they get very near to their due date. Either way, the good news is that the swelling is just water retention and should disappear completely after the baby is born.

Have I had any swelling in my hands or feet—or any place else? Have I made my doctor aware of this swelling?

_____

_____

What precautions am I taking to avoid swelling? Am I trying to stay off my feet more and modifying my diet to avoid salty foods?

_____

_____

_____

How would I describe my baby's movement during this time? When is he most active? What seems to prompt him to move around more?

_____

_____

WEEK 30—SoulWise

Have you thought about what your parenting style will be? As I said earlier, it's a good idea to watch other parents with their children. It will show you many ways that you do—and don't!—want to raise your own child. Also think about your own—and your partner's—upbringing and how this might be a factor in your own parenting. If you had very strict, authoritarian parents, will this make you authoritarian? Or will you rebel against your own upbringing and be permissive? If you felt neglected in your home, you may be pledging to be more attentive to your child than your own parents were to you. There is a lot to think about because a lot of factors will influence the kind of parent you will be. Ultimately, you will be able to make deliberate and reasoned choices for the way you will parent your child.

What five words describe the parenting style that I hope to have?

_____

_____

How would I describe my parents' parenting style? What things will I do the same and what will I do differently?

_____

_____

_____

How does my partner describe his parents' style? Does he wish to parent the way they did or differently?

_____

_____

_____

Have my partner and I discussed and compared our ideal parenting styles? Do we seem to be alike or have major differences? How can we come to share a mutual vision?

_____

_____

_____

AMONG THIS WEEK'S WONDERS:

1:

Your baby's brain now looks like a person's, with lots of wrinkles!

2:

Baby is now taking in all of the calcium, protein, and iron you give him.

3:

Baby's bone marrow takes over the production of red blood cells.

4:

Your baby's eyes can now open and close.

5:

The hair on your baby's body has started to disappear, but he may have a full head of hair.

THREE THINGS TO DO THIS WEEK:

1. *Make a list of questions to ask my doctor at the next visit.*
2. *Discuss with my partner how our parenting styles are alike and different, how each complements the other style, and what our mutual goals as parents are.*
3. _____

Week 31

Becoming a Little Absentminded

Being pregnant can be quite a distraction. When you're supposed to be

thinking about your next meeting at work, you might

instead find yourself thinking about your baby.

Word to the Mother-to-Be: As you come closer to your baby's birth, chances are you find yourself thinking about her more and more. You're busy making decisions about whether you'll return to work, and if so, what your child-care arrangements will be. You're planning the nursery and worrying about labor. If this isn't your first child, you're wondering how your other child or children will adjust. And on and on the list goes. Is it any wonder, then, that you suddenly find yourself being a little absentminded or forgetful?

It's not uncommon for pregnant women to complain of suddenly being absentminded and having trouble concentrating. If you're experiencing this symptom of pregnancy, the first thing you should know is that it's okay and it won't last past your pregnancy—except, perhaps, on those days following particularly sleepless nights. So relax. Accept this absentmindedness as just one more way that you are sacrificing your own comfort for your child's. You can also find simple tricks for getting around the problem of forgetfulness or absentmindedness. For example, start writing little reminders to yourself, take on fewer responsibilities, and ask others to remind you of tasks you have in common. Another way to deal with this issue is to try to be as relaxed about it as possible. If you feel tense or anxious about this sudden loss of focus, chances are you'll only end up more distracted and unable to focus.

WEEK 31 — BODYWISE

For health reasons, now is the time when you should stop air travel. If you travel a lot as part of your occupation, it is important to send someone in your place or put off trips until you return from maternity leave. Sitting for long periods on a cramped plane and the changes in altitude can be harmful to your body and your baby. And, of course, as you get closer to your delivery date, you'll want to be as close as possible to your own doctor and hospital. If you're considering air travel at this time, it may be appropriate to reconsider. Be sure to talk to your doctor first.

If I have to travel for work, am I concerned that my colleagues will not be understanding of my need to forego upcoming trips? Am I comfortable accepting their lack of understanding to put my own and my baby's health first?

_____

_____

_____

Have I been feeling absentminded or forgetful lately? What are my techniques for dealing with this condition?

_____

_____

_____

What questions do I have for my doctor this week?

_____

_____

_____

WEEK 31—SoulWise

No doubt you've heard that raising a child is quite an expensive endeavor. As you prepare for your child's birth, also prepare for your financial security. If you haven't been very good with handling money in the past, you may want to consult a financial advisor. You'll need to consider important questions. For example, if you're considering being a stay-at-home mom or only working part-time, how will your family manage on a single or reduced income? Can you afford daycare? How much will health insurance cost with another family member on the plan? Getting smart about your finances is an important way to ensure your family's well-being. Get a plan together now for eliminating needless expenses, reducing your debt, and building a secure financial future for your family.

How would I rate my financial health on a scale of 1 to 10 (with 10 being very healthy)? Why did I give myself this score?

_____

_____

Do I plan to leave my job or cut back on hours? If so, how well will our family manage on less income?

_____

_____

_____

Have my partner and I discussed our financial concerns? What things are we in agreement about? What areas of disagreement do we have? How can we resolve them?

_____

_____

_____

AMONG THIS WEEK'S WONDERS:

1:

Baby's growth will slow down a bit. However, she should still gain
two more pounds before birth.

2:

The baby's irises can now dilate and contract in response to light.

3:

All of baby's systems continue to become more complex.

4:

Your baby now has the same brain waves as an adult.

5:

If your baby is a boy, his testes begin to descend from the body cavity to the scrotum.

6:

Deposits of white fat underneath the skin make baby's skin pink instead of red.

THREE THINGS TO DO THIS WEEK:

1. *Reschedule any travel plans I had for the next few months.*
2. *Prepare a budget reflecting my adjusted income and expenses after the baby is born.*
3. _____

Week 32

Feeling Showered with Love and Friendship

My shower made me realize how lucky I am to have

such wonderful friends and family with whom I can share

the frustrations and joys of motherhood.

A *Word to the Mother-to-Be:* If you haven't already been thinking about your baby shower and registering for the items you need for your baby, now is a great time to start. I loved my baby shower. Of course I got many great gifts—some cute and frilly things, and some practical essentials—but the gifts weren't the only reason I loved my shower. Instead, it was the great atmosphere where everything was about babies—mine and other moms'. It was fun talking to all of my experienced mommy friends about their parenting experiences. It was like going to camp and swapping stories around the campfire, only the fire was really a mound of pastel ribbons! Spending those few hours immersed in chatter about pregnancy and infant care made me realize I had a whole network of experts to turn to on occasions when I felt uncertain or frustrated. All the books I'd been reading told me I must be willing to call on my friends for help after I get home from the hospital. My baby shower made me realize how many good friends I had who would be willing to provide insight and support when I need it. That alone made this baby shower business well worth it. Of course, all the great gifts I received weren't bad either.

So this week, as you look forward to your baby shower with anticipation, think about all the wonderful gifts you'll receive—the ones wrapped in pretty ribbons and the ones that are harder to measure: the affection and caring of your close friends and your family.

WEEK 32—BODYWISE

Around week 32 you may start experiencing Braxton Hicks contractions, also known as false labor. These contractions give your uterus a chance to practice contracting and relaxing, just as it does during delivery. Braxton Hicks contractions tend to be felt earlier and more intensely by women who have experienced a prior pregnancy, and can sometimes start as early as the twentieth week of pregnancy. These contractions (unlike those for birth) usually don't hurt, but you may experience them more and more often as you get closer to your delivery date. Although Braxton Hicks contractions are not strong enough to deliver your baby, they may get the pre-birth process of effacement and early dilation started, thus giving you a bit of a head start for your delivery. To relieve the discomfort of the contractions, try changing your position—lie down if you've been moving around, or sit if you've been walking or standing. If you experience these contractions very frequently (more than four an hour), report them to your doctor.

Am I experiencing any contractions yet? If so, what do they feel like?

_____

_____

_____

Have I discussed any contractions or other unusual sensations with my doctor? What advice has he or she given?

_____

_____

_____

How confident am I that I'll know when the contractions I experience are the real thing?

_____

_____

WEEK 32—SOULWISE

My shower made me realize that my partner and I aren't the only ones who will love our baby dearly. She's going to be lucky to have so many people who care about her and love her! As you think about your pregnancy and anticipate the birth of your child, think about all the people who have given you special love and attention during your pregnancy, and the people who will be an important part of your child's life. Be sure to let them know how important they are to you and how much their support and friendship mean to you. If you've felt like the center of the universe at times because of all the concern and attention that has been lavished on you during your pregnancy, be sure not to become self-centered. Instead, think of the people around you who have shared in the joys (and aches and pains) of your pregnancy, and who will be an important part of your family's life after your child is born. Be grateful for having them in your life, and be sure to let them know how you feel.

What family members do I expect to be a special part of my child's life?

_____

_____

_____

What friends do I hope to have in my child's life as he grows?

_____

_____

What friendships have been most important to me during my pregnancy? Have I thanked those people and let them know how important they are to me?

_____

_____

_____

AMONG THIS WEEK'S WONDERS:

1:
All five of baby's senses are working now.

2:
Your baby develops his papillary reflex, which means the iris of the eye opens wider when lighting is dim and gets smaller when the light is bright.

3:
Your baby's toenails will become fully formed.

4:
Baby's brain is now pushing against his skull.

THREE THINGS TO DO THIS WEEK:

1. Speak to my doctor if I feel like I'm having any contractions.
2. Write a letter to a special friend to thank this person for his or her support during my pregnancy.
3. _____

Week 33

How Big Will My Baby Be?

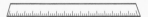

If you're worried about having a large baby—and a challenging delivery—
talk to your doctor about how he or she will decide
whether it's time to deliver by cesarean.

A *Word to the Mother-to-Be:* By now, you should be gaining about a pound a week. If your weight gain so far has been on the high side, you may be starting to worry that you are going to have a large baby—and a more challenging delivery. However, your higher-than-average weight gain doesn't automatically mean that your baby will be larger than average. Other factors will also influence your baby's size. For example, if you were born small, your baby is likely to be small, too.

At the time of delivery, if the medical practitioner determines that a baby is too large to fit through the mother's pelvis, chances are he or she would still allow natural labor. However, this labor trial will be carefully monitored, and if labor doesn't progress as it should, the doctor may choose to proceed with a cesarean delivery.

If your doctor confirms that your baby will be larger than average (or perhaps average size but still too large in proportion to your pelvis), discuss with your doctor the approach that will be used in the delivery room. Find out your doctor's philosophy in such cases, and remember that you don't have to be a silent participant in the decision making. Let your doctor know how you feel about a cesarean and whether you would be more comfortable moving ahead with one earlier in the delivery process if labor doesn't progress.

Week 33—Body Wise

Finding a comfortable position is probably becoming more and more difficult these days. When you sit, you may find that you are shifting frequently just to take the pressure off the part of your body you're sitting on. Standing for long periods is usually out of the question. And you'll probably wake up several times during the night when an arm or leg falls asleep under the weight of your body and you need to turn over. And, of course, there are the bathroom trips. Now that baby is permanently planted, it seems, right on your bladder, you're probably getting up several times a night just to find relief. Make sure you have a nightlight on so you don't stumble over something in the dark.

Is it getting harder to stay comfortable for long periods in a chair? Is it more difficult to sit through a movie or spend long periods at a desk?

_____

_____

_____

What parts of my body are the most sore—my feet, my back, or my belly? Or do I just feel sore all over?

_____

_____

_____

Do I have reason to think that my baby will be larger than average at birth? What has my doctor said about my baby's size?

_____

_____

WEEK 33—SOULWISE

By this point in your pregnancy, you've probably had the experience of dealing with another expectant mom who seems to be in competition over who'll have the bigger baby, whose baby kicks more, who is up more times during the night, and so on. This mom is probably also the one who'll be comparing her child to everyone else's— wanting to know which child crawled first, walked first, and said her first word earlier. Clearly, this is not the ideal way to experience pregnancy or motherhood, which should be about a mother's love for her child and the child's individual development. If you find yourself around a hypercompetitive mom, especially if you're the type to be sensitive and worry about your own baby's development, discourage further competition by sharing as little as possible. Better yet, avoid such company and focus instead on your baby and her development milestones.

How do I respond when other expectant moms compare our pregnancies? Am I easily made to worry about my baby's development?

_____

_____

_____

How should I respond when another expectant mom makes competitive remarks about our pregnancies? Am I able to think about the days ahead with my own little baby, and smile and let it go?

_____

_____

_____

✎ *Do I have a tendency to mentally compare my own pregnancy to other pregnant moms'*
experiences? Is this a productive habit or one I should give up? Why?

_____

_____

_____

AMONG THIS WEEK'S WONDERS:

1:

Rapid brain growth continues this week, increasing the baby's head size
by 3/8 of an inch this week.

2:

Baby's skin is getting pinker and less transparent as fat continues
to develop underneath.

3:

Fat continues to accumulate, turning the baby's skin color from red to pink.

4:

Your baby weighs about 3 pounds and is almost 15 inches long.

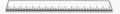

THREE THINGS TO DO THIS WEEK:

1.   Make arrangements to visit the hospital where I will be delivering, if I haven't done so
     already.
2.   Make a decision to avoid the company of those who are too competitive when it
     comes to pregnancy or parenting, and be sure I don't behave that way myself.
3.   _____

Week 34

Baby Is Preparing for Descent

By now, chances are you find yourself waking up in the night

thinking about your baby.

A *Word to the Mother-to-Be:* Sometime between weeks 32 and 36, most babies settle into a head-down position. However, some babies will still be in the breech position as these weeks pass. When a fetus is still in the breech position near term, the obstetrician may attempt to turn him around. This procedure is called external cephalic version (ECV), and involves applying manual pressure to the mother's abdomen to gently, with the guidance of ultrasound, try to shift the baby into the head-down position. This procedure is typically performed at about 37 weeks. During ECV, it's crucial to monitor the baby to ensure that the umbilical cord isn't accidentally compressed or the placenta disturbed.

Successful ECV can reduce the need for a cesarean delivery. (Occasionally, the fetus will revert back to the breech position after successful ECV.) Only a physician who has been trained in ECV—and cesarean delivery—can perform the procedure.

If your baby is one of the 3 to 4 percent in breech position at birth, discuss the delivery with your doctor. You may still be able to have a vaginal delivery, but a cesarean is also a possibility at this point. Be sure to talk to your doctor ahead of time and be informed of how he or she will proceed if the baby remains in the breech position.

WEEK 34—BODYWISE

At this point in your pregnancy, you are gaining about a pound a week. All the symptoms you've been experiencing in the past few weeks are likely to be magnified. You are more tired, your belly is itchier than it's been, you're sleeping even less at night, and so on. Another symptom of late pregnancy that you may now be experiencing is the leakage of colostrum from your breasts. Colostrum is a pre-milk substance. It is richer in protein and lower in fat and milk sugar than breast milk. It contains antibodies that may be important to protecting the baby against disease. Colostrum continues to be produced for the first three or four days after delivery, when milk production begins. Some women do not have any noticeable colostrum before delivery, so don't feel anxious if you do not.

How am I feeling this week? What symptoms am I experiencing most strongly?

_____

_____

_____

Have I noticed any colostrum leakage? When did this first occur?

_____

_____

_____

Besides my protruding belly, what are the most visible changes I notice about my appearance?

_____

_____

_____

WEEK 34—SOULWISE

Restless nights are a routine part of pregnancy by week 34. Considering your frequent visits to the bathroom, achy back, and shortness of breath, sleeping for more than two hours at a stretch can seem like a blessing. But those physical symptoms are probably not the only thing keeping you from a sound sleep. Chances are, by now, you find yourself waking up in the night thinking about your baby. There is so much to wonder about, prepare for, and go over in your mind. When you find yourself waking up at night and wondering (and maybe worrying) about your baby and all the responsibility you will soon be facing, focus on all the wonderful ways you've cared for your child so far, and affirm that your love for him will guide you even when you face difficult moments. And when you're just too excited to go to sleep, remember that soon you'll be facing many feeding calls in the night, so curl up under the covers now and sleep while you can.

When I wake during the night, what thoughts tend to preoccupy me and keep me awake?

_____

_____

_____

In what ways do I feel most prepared for my baby's birth? In what ways do I worry about not being prepared enough?

_____

_____

_____

Five words I would use to describe my feelings when I think about my child's birth are:

_____

_____

AMONG THIS WEEK'S WONDERS:

1:
If your baby were born this week, he is mature enough to survive outside your body.

2:
Your baby will grow another half inch this week.

3:
Babies' eyes are blue at this point and won't develop their true color
until three months after birth.

4:
Baby's own immune system is beginning to function.

5:
The baby's fingernails are getting long, and may even require a trim after birth.

6:
Although most of baby's parts are fully formed, the brain continues
its critical development.

THREE THINGS TO DO THIS WEEK:

1. *Prepare a list of names and numbers of people to call when I go into labor and for phone calls from the hospital when my baby is born. (You can use page 175 in the "Planning for Baby" section to write these down.)*
2. *Talk to my partner about how he is feeling now that the baby's birth is near.*
3. _____

Week 35

Packed and Ready to Go

When baby decides she is ready, you need to be ready, too.

A **Word to the Mother-to-Be:** Now that you are in week 35 of your pregnancy, your baby is about 18 inches long and weighs about 5½ pounds, and can see and hear. Most of the baby's systems are well developed, and if born now, she has an excellent chance of survival with few complications.

Now that your baby is just about ready to make her entry into the world, it's time to prepare yourself for your trip to the hospital. You have probably made most of your other preparations by now. You have the nursery set up, the car seat installed, and a six-month supply of diapers stacked in the closet. Don't overlook packing for the hospital. Trust me, if you go into labor at 3 A.M., you don't want to be running around trying to figure out what to throw in a shopping bag! Get out an attractive carrying case or piece of luggage and get started. Treat yourself to a couple of pretty pajamas or nightgowns—and make sure they button down the front for easy access if you plan to breastfeed. Take your toiletries, of course. And don't forget going-home outfits for you and the baby. And pack anything you'll want for the delivery room, like a tape of special music and your camera. Once your bag is packed, you can relax knowing that no matter when or at what time your baby is ready, you'll be ready too! You can use the list on pages 173–174 in the "Planning for Baby" section as a general guide for the types of things you might want to pack.

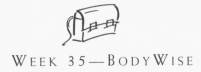

WEEK 35—BODYWISE

As you approach your ninth month, your doctor will probably be seeing you week-ly and monitoring you more closely. He or she might begin regular checks of your cervix some time in the next few weeks for signs of effacement (thinning) and dila-tion. In addition, your doctor may also begin monitoring any contractions you might be having, checking the baby's position to see if she's dropped, as well as assessing your weight gain and any swelling you're experiencing, monitoring your blood pres-sure, and checking your urine for sugar and protein. As you approach your due date, it is important to be under the close care of your doctor, so be sure to keep all your appointments and let your doctor know if anything feels different or if you are experiencing any new symptoms.

How am I feeling now that I'm in my thirty-fifth week? How frequently am I seeing my doctor?

_____

_____

_____

What does my doctor check during my appointments? Has he or she commented on any issues, such as swelling or my blood pressure?

_____

_____

_____

Has my baby dropped? Is she positioning herself for birth yet?

_____

_____

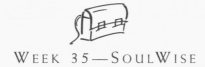

WEEK 35—SoulWise

During my pregnancy, I worried and wondered about how I would do as a parent. I knew I would love my child, but wondered if I had all the skills I needed to be the best parent possible. I don't think that being a good parent is something that we just instinctively know. It's important to observe other parents, ask for advice, read books, take classes—do whatever it takes to learn good parenting skills. Although loving our children usually comes naturally, we will still face many situations that we won't be sure how to handle. Parenting is sometimes a learn-as-you-go task, but the more you know up front the better.

Do I have a friend or family member whom I consider to be a good role model for parenting? Have I sought out his or her advice?

_____

_____

_____

Have I considered taking a class to learn good parenting skills? Where might such classes become available? Can I convince my partner to attend with me?

_____

_____

_____

Have I asked my mother about what she learned in parenting my siblings and me? What helpful advice was she able to offer?

_____

_____

_____

AMONG THIS WEEK'S WONDERS:

1:
Baby weighs about 5½ pounds now and is almost 18 inches long.

2:
The fat accumulation plumps up baby's arms and legs.

3:
Baby is big enough to take up most of the uterus, allowing less room for movement.

4:
The testes have completed their descent in males.

5:
Your baby could begin dropping into the pelvic region this week,
although not all babies do.

6:
The baby is storing extra nutrients from you in case she is born a little early
since her digestive tract won't be completely efficient yet.

7:
Baby is storing more iron from your body for use in the first few months after birth.

THREE THINGS TO DO THIS WEEK:

1. *Write down any questions I have for my doctor and record the results of any additional testing.*
2. *Study up on parenting skills: Read books, attend classes, and consult with other parents.*
3. _____

Week 36

Has My Baby "Dropped"?

*You're definitely in the home stretch now—your baby
is almost ready for birth.*

A Word to the Mother-to-Be: Welcome to the ninth month. You're definitely in the home stretch. With just four weeks to go, your baby is almost ready for birth. He could drop into the birth canal at any time now. Dropping, also called "lightening," occurs when the baby descends into the pelvic cavity. For women who have had children previously, dropping is less likely to occur before labor begins. For first-time mothers, dropping can occur up to four weeks before the due date. However, it is also possible for first-time mothers to go into labor without dropping.

It is quite likely that when your baby drops you will know it. Your belly will seem lower and tilted farther forward. Another indication that your baby has dropped may be the sudden release of pressure on your diaphragm, making it easier to breathe. On the downside, however, you may also notice increased pressure on your bladder and pelvic joints, causing increased frequency of urination and uncomfortable or difficult mobility. Remember, though, that it's also possible for dropping to occur without your realizing it. This is especially likely if you were carrying low to begin with.

Remember that whether your baby has dropped or not is not an indication of how close you are to delivering. There is no way to know that for certain until you go into labor or your water breaks (or you go far enough past your due date that your doctor must induce labor).

WEEK 36—BODYWISE

Don't be shocked if you gain more weight than expected due to fluid retention. On the other hand, you may not gain very much now, as your baby's growth slows and you feel less desire to eat. Even if your appetite has decreased, however, be sure to maintain a higher-than-normal calorie count, by eating healthy and nutritious food. As you've done so far, continue to avoid junk calories. Use your calorie intake efficiently, instead, making every calorie work for your baby's healthy development.

How am I feeling? Does my body feel like the baby has dropped—that is, is there more pressure on my bladder and pelvis but less on my diaphragm and stomach?

_____

_____

_____

What do I weigh now? How much weight have I gained so far?

_____

_____

_____

Am I worried about getting the weight off after I have the baby? Do I hope to return to my original weight? Is that realistic?

_____

_____

_____

WEEK 36—SoulWise

Watching baby-food commercials or flipping through parenting magazines gives one the impression that all babies are simply adorable and are always smiling. They make parenting look easy. Who wouldn't want such an adorable and happy child at home? But, of course, the reality is that, just like us, babies have their good days and their "off" days. On some days, your baby might fuss, cry for no apparent reason, and just find it difficult to go to sleep. Even though you'll love your baby with all your heart, there will be days when you'll wish you were lying on a beach in Aruba—alone! When your baby is having a bad day, remember that it will pass. Focus on his beautiful smile and how much you love this little soul, and how grateful you are to provide the love and comfort your little one needs in adjusting to his new world.

How do I think I will cope when my baby is having an "off" day? What skills do I have that will help me cope with those situations?

_____

_____

_____

Whom can I turn to for encouragement when it feels like my baby just won't stop fussing or crying? Do I trust myself to care for the needs of my newborn?

_____

_____

_____

Do I expect my partner to be supportive and helpful in caring for our baby, even when he is fussy? How can I help my partner to be an involved and hands-on parent?

_____

_____

_____

_____

_____

AMONG THIS WEEK'S WONDERS:

1:

Your baby's growth is now beginning to slow. He is conserving his energy
for the birthing process.

2:

Increased fat deposits cause those adorable dimples in baby's knees and elbows.

3:

Baby's gums have ridges.

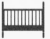

THREE THINGS TO DO THIS WEEK:

1. _Sign up for a baby-care class._
2. _Work on controlling any angry or impatient tendencies I might have so that I can handle the stresses of a fussy baby._
3. _____

Week 37

Counting Down

After eight months of physical, emotional, and mental preparation

for a baby, the last month can often feel slow and long.

A Word to the Mother-to-Be: By week 37, you are probably feeling quite impatient to have your baby. Not only are you tired of being tired, and of all the aches and pains, but you probably can't wait to meet your baby. By this time in your pregnancy, it's natural to start feeling impatient and restless. Many women also find that they have increased mood changes or more intense feelings of excitement or anxiety. It's also not uncommon during the ninth month for an expectant mom to find that she is dreaming or thinking about the baby more than ever. After eight months of physical, emotional, and mental preparation for a baby—not to mention practical preparations, such as fixing up the nursery and buying essential equipment—the last month can easily leave you feeling like you're so close to the finish mark, but still just shy of it.

If you find yourself feeling impatient for your pregnancy to be over so that you can finally see and hold your baby, look for productive ways to fill your time. For example, you can pick out your birth announcement, be sure you have thank-you cards on hand, and stock up on any odds and ends you haven't yet purchased or received. Even better than doing chores would be to give yourself some pre-baby treats. For example, plan lunch dates with your mom, sisters, or girlfriends; finish reading that novel you started that will surely start to collect dust after your baby is born; and catch a movie or two at the theater while you can still get a night (or even an afternoon) out.

WEEK 37—BODYWISE

Now is not the time to be superwoman. I read about a woman who tried to cook the entire Thanksgiving dinner in her ninth month of pregnancy! Of course, she had committed to doing this chore three months before the holiday, when she was considerably lighter on her feet. She only made it as far as the mashed potatoes. Fortunately, her relatives took charge and handled the rest of the menu. If you have a big occasion looming and you're just not feeling up to handling it, ask for help or turn the work over to somebody else! Listen to your body and avoid doing more than you can comfortably handle. Give someone a chance to lend a helping hand. You might even discover that your husband has been hiding some useful skills that will come in handy now and in the future.

Have I made any time commitments that I'm now dreading because I don't feel up to them? What will I do to resolve this dilemma?

_____

_____

Whom can I count on to help me out if I can't handle as much as I usually do?

_____

_____

Have I asked my partner to give me a hand in household responsibilities that I normally take on myself, such as shopping or laundry? What has been his response?

_____

_____

WEEK 37—SoulWise

As you look forward to your baby's birth, chances are you spend quite a bit of time imagining what she'll be like and all the ways in which you'll be a great mother to her. Now is a good opportunity to think about traditions you want to share with your child. Think about traditions, or even heirlooms, that have been handed down in your family that have been important to you. For example, you may recall your mother's or father's storytelling when you were a child, or you may recall a special holiday custom your family kept up for all the years you were growing. Consider which of your own traditions you want to pass down to your child and maintain in your own family. Also think about new family traditions you would like to create for your own family. This can be a marvelous gift to give to your child.

What holiday traditions do I treasure most and want to pass on to my child?

_____

_____

_____

Does my partner have any family traditions he is eager to maintain in our family?

_____

_____

_____

What new traditions or customs do I want to create and make a part of my child's life?

_____

_____

_____

✐ *In what ways do I feel my child's life will be enriched by sharing in family traditions?*

_____

_____

_____

AMONG THIS WEEK'S WONDERS:

1:

Baby weighs around 6½ pounds now, but her growth has slowed down quite a bit.

2:

Your baby's grip is getting even firmer.

3:

Baby consistently turns toward sources of light.

4:

The baby practices breathing movements preparing for life outside the womb.

THREE THINGS TO DO THIS WEEK:

1. *Rethink any commitments I have coming up and ask for help if the work is more than I can handle.*
2. *Talk to my partner about the family traditions we'd like to share—and create—for our family.*
3. _____

Week 38

Leaving the Old Life Behind

Will you be a working mom or a stay-at-home mom? Remember that
you have the wisdom you need to do what will be for the best.

A *Word to the Mother-to-Be:* If you'd been working during your pregnancy, you're probably on maternity leave by now. Have you given much thought to when you might return to work, or to how you will adjust your work schedule to accommodate your new responsibilities? Have you decided whether you will return to work or be a full-time mom? Sometimes financial reasons make it a necessity to return to work. At other times, a woman may choose to make work and family a part of her life.

Deciding whether to be a full-time mom, to work part-time, or to return to a full-time job is a personal decision, one based on a variety of factors. The decision you make has to be right for you and for your family. It should not be influenced by social or peer expectations or by the attitudes of other people. Only you, together with your partner, can decide what is best for your family. And only you can fully know what it will mean for you to give up either full-time parenting or your work life. Weigh the options, consider the pros and cons, and think honestly about how you will ultimately feel about the decision you make. The important thing is to make the choice that will give you satisfaction and fulfillment and that will help you meet the goals you have set for yourself—even if those goals have changed since you became pregnant.

Week 38 — BodyWise

By now, you're probably on the lookout for the onset of labor. Before labor begins, however, you might also experience pre-labor symptoms. These might precede labor by as much as a month—or by only a few hours. Signs of pre-labor include the baby dropping; sensations of increased pressure on the pelvis and rectum; a noticeable increase or decrease in energy level; intensified Braxton Hicks contractions; and pink or bloody discharge, caused by ruptured capillaries as the cervix dilates. When you visit your doctor, he or she will be able to identify some of these pre-labor symptoms if they have occurred. Most of these symptoms are not a definite indication that labor is about to start. However, if you see a pink discharge, this may be a sign that you will be going into labor within the next day or so. Be prepared to call your doctor when this happens.

How am I feeling? Have I experienced any pre-labor symptoms?

_____

_____

_____

Have I been gaining weight during the ninth month, or has my weight remained the same or decreased?

_____

_____

Have I noticed a change in my energy level?

_____

_____

_____

✎ *In what ways do I feel different this month than I did last month?*

_____

_____

_____

☀

WEEK 38—SOULWISE

Making major life decisions—such as whether to change jobs, get married, or have a baby—takes courage. Sometimes it's hard to know what to do. You hope for a sign that will tell you which path to take. If pregnancy and the prospect of motherhood—or another child in the family—has made you question whether to choose career and motherhood or to give up the former for the latter, you may well be experiencing conflicting emotions over the decision. But whatever you choose, remember that your goal is to be the best mother to your children you can possibly be. And only you can know whether you will achieve that by being a full-time mom or by being a working mom and a source of financial support to your family. Trust yourself to make the decision that will be best for you and your family.

✎ *Do I feel conflicted about any choices I've made or have yet to make about my future work plans? What conflicting emotions do I feel?*

_____

_____

_____

✎ *Have I gathered all the information that I can about my options? Have I ruled out anything based on this information?*

_____

_____

_____

Have I discussed my feelings and preferences with my partner? What does he feel would be the right thing to do? Am I sensitive to his concerns about my decision?

_____

_____

_____

AMONG THIS WEEK'S WONDERS:

1:

Meconium—cells and waste from the liver, gall bladder, and pancreas—is accumulating in the baby's intestines. (Baby has his first bowel movement.)

2:

Baby's toenails now extend to the end of his toes.

3:

A baby girl's labia majora have formed.

4:

Baby may be gaining an ounce a day now.

5:

The circumference of the baby's head and abdomen are about the same.

THREE THINGS TO DO THIS WEEK:

1. *If I'm still wondering whether I will return to work after my baby's birth, take time to carefully consider my options and the pros and cons of each choice.*
2. *Research and consider options I haven't thought of before, such as working part-time.*
3. _____

Week 39

Is It Time to Call the Doctor?

Weary as you may feel, it's time to be thankful for a baby
who has gone to term.

A **Word to the Mother-to-Be:** Now that we've covered pre-labor (in week 38), let's talk about real labor symptoms. Labor has probably started if you experience any of the following: intensified contractions that persist even if you change position or engage in mild activity; the contractions become more frequent and occur at regularly spaced intervals; the pain begins in your lower back and moves to your abdomen; the painfulness of the contractions intensifies progressively; the membrane ruptures (also known as water breaking). Note, however, that although the contractions generally accelerate in frequency and become progressively more painful, they do at times slow down or become less painful. The key is to feel an overall acceleration in frequency and intensity. Anytime you're in doubt, it doesn't hurt to call your doctor.

As you wait for the first signs of real labor, try to just relax. You may be feeling impatient, but at this point, it really won't be much longer before you're calling your doctor and heading for the hospital.

WEEK 39—BODYWISE

By now, you're probably feeling huge. Even the smallest task may be leaving you feeling tired. As the baby settles into your pelvis (lightening, or dropping) you may also be finding yourself getting a little clumsy because your center of gravity has shifted, making you feel off-balance. The good news is that by now you can breathe more easily because your uterus isn't pressing on your diaphragm. However, it may now be pushing on your bladder, forcing you to run to the bathroom at twenty-minute intervals.

Have I had any symptoms that I thought were the start of labor? What symptoms did I experience?

_____

_____

_____

Am I afraid of going into labor? Looking forward to it? What are my thoughts now, knowing that it could happen at any time?

_____

_____

_____

Is my partner anxious about me going into labor? Is he on edge or calm about it?

_____

_____

_____

Overall, how do I feel this week?

_____

_____

_____

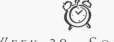

WEEK 39—SoulWise

It's a waiting game now. You could go into labor two hours from now, or it might not happen for three more weeks! Either way, you can now feel thankful that your baby has gone to term and you can feel good about all the care you've taken to nurture her throughout your pregnancy.

Do I feel really anxious to know when I'll go into labor, or am I pretty calm about the whole thing?

_____

_____

_____

How many people have called me today to say, "You haven't had that baby yet?" What is my usual response?

_____

_____

_____

How is my body holding up? Am I tired, uncomfortable, or feeling pretty good?

_____

_____

_____

In what ways do I feel good about the way I've mothered my baby throughout this pregnancy?

_____

_____

THREE THINGS TO DO THIS WEEK:

1. *Have the list of names and numbers of people to call when I go into labor and for phone calls from the hospital when my baby is born handy (see page 175 in the "Planning for Baby" section).*

2. *If it's not already done, be sure my bag is packed and ready to go (see the list on p. 173 in the "Planning for Baby" section).*

3. _____

Week 40

It's My Due Date!

Even if your due date comes and goes and you're still waiting, rest assured

that it really is just a matter of days before you will have your baby.

A *Word to the Mother-to-Be:* This week marks your due date. You are in your fortieth week of pregnancy. It has been approximately thirty-eight weeks since your baby's conception, and your baby is now full-term. Keep in mind, though, that your due date is just an estimate (perhaps thinking of it as a "due week" will create more realistic expectations), so don't be impatient as you wait for that specific day, and don't be disappointed if that day comes and goes and you're still at home. Also remember that you aren't officially considered past due until you've hit forty-two weeks of pregnancy. At that point, your doctor will probably discuss labor induction with you. Some obstetricians opt for induction by forty-one weeks. In gauging when to induce, your doctor's main concern will be how well your baby is doing.

So now, although you may feel discouraged and be wondering if the pregnancy will ever end, you can rest assured that at the longest, it will be just another two weeks. But that is an extreme estimate; only 10 percent of pregnancies go to forty-two weeks. You can rest assured that it really is just a matter of days at this point.

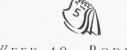

WEEK 40—BODYWISE

Amazingly, doctors still don't really know what tells the body to begin labor. Does the message come from your baby? Does your body decide? Does it have something to do with your hormones or the baby's pressure on your body? The answer isn't clear. Similarly, some women's cervixes will begin to dilate several weeks in advance while others don't dilate until right before they deliver. Your body is unique. One thing is sure, though: It will only be a matter of days before your body will begin labor. Treat your body well, and it will soon give you the sign that the time has arrived.

How am I feeling? Have I noticed any signs of labor yet? What does my doctor say about my readiness?

_____

_____

_____

What is my gut feeling about when I'll go into labor? Do I think I'll have the baby this week, or do I not feel physically ready yet?

_____

_____

_____

How do I envision my labor starting? Do I think my water will break? Will I start having contractions? What scenario plays out in my mind when I picture the start of labor?

_____

_____

_____

Am I feeling anxious and impatient or relaxed?

_____

_____

_____

WEEK 40—SoulWise

As you wait for labor to start, relax and do your best to stay comfortable. Stay busy by spending time with people whose company you enjoy. When your partner is at work, invite your mom, sister, or a close friend to spend time with you. Spending time chatting and laughing will be a good way to get your mind off the waiting, and will keep you cheerful when you might be feeling like you've lost patience with being tired. Do your best to keep your spirits up whenever you start to feel anxious about labor, or about going too far past your due date.

Do I feel stressed or anxious? What helps me cope with these moments?

_____

_____

_____

What does my doctor say about when he or she thinks I will deliver and the baby's size? Do I consider this to be good news or bad news? Why?

_____

_____

_____

🖉 *How am I feeling during my fortieth week?*

_____

_____

_____

THREE THINGS TO DO THIS WEEK:

1.   *Relax! Do what I can to decrease anxiety.*
2.   *Take short walks to stay in shape and eliminate stress.*
3.   _____

Weeks 41+

Going Beyond Full-Term

Can you believe you're still pregnant? Perhaps your baby just wanted

a little more time with you all to herself!

A **Word to the Mother-to-Be:** If you're still reading this, it means you've gone past your due date and are now entering your forty-first week. Can you believe you're still pregnant? Your baby just wanted a little more time with you all to herself! After all, the world's a pretty overwhelming place to a baby who's known nothing but the perfect comfort of your womb. She had the comforting sounds of your heart and your voice to make her feel cozy, and all her needs were met on demand, thanks to the wonders of your own body. No wonder she's reluctant to make the transition!

As for you, of course, it's a different story! You are eager and ready to meet this new member of your family. You are also ready to quit hauling around your big belly and the extra weight. That is completely understandable. Every mother who has gone past week 40 has experienced some frustration at having to go on waiting. But while you wait, take time to congratulate yourself on a job well-done. Look back on all you've done to care for your baby while you carried her in your womb, and let that affirm for you the many ways in which you will love, nurture, and care for your baby when she is born and as she grows.

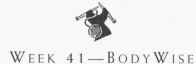

Week 41 — BodyWise

Do you feel like the doctor's office is now your home away from home? You've been going there for months now, and the visits have only escalated as you've gotten closer to—and now past!—your due date. You're certain that you could dial the office phone number with your eyes closed! Well, be thankful the doctor is taking good care of you because you'll soon be relying on him or her to bring your precious baby into the world, as well as to make sure that you recover fully and completely after your baby's birth. And remember, before long, you'll be trading in your visits to the OB-GYN for those to the pediatrician.

🖉 *When was my last visit to the doctor? What was his or her advice?*

_____

_____

_____

🖉 *Has the doctor suggested any techniques to hurry things along? Has he or she given me a deadline before I'll be induced?*

_____

_____

_____

🖉 *How is my body holding up now that I'm post-term? Is it giving me signs that it's more than ready to birth this baby?*

_____

_____

_____

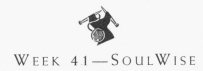

Week 41—SoulWise

Sure, your body is more than ready, but your heart and soul are anxious, too. When will this baby be born? What's taking so long? It doesn't help that friends and family members are constantly calling to ask, "Are you in labor yet?" Although they mean well, it's tempting to say, "Don't call me; I'll call you when it happens!" But don't let other people's impatience or good-natured questioning bother you. Soon you (or more likely your partner) will be calling them to announce the news of your baby's birth. Enjoy the attentiveness people are showing you. It's a sign of their affection for you and of their eager anticipation of your baby's birth.

Did I ever imagine I'd still be waiting for my baby's arrival at forty-one-plus weeks? How do I feel about that?

_____

_____

_____

Am I worried about being late, or relaxed knowing that the best thing I can do is to remain calm?

_____

_____

_____

Have friends and family members been calling for updates on my progress? Do I enjoy receiving their calls or feel irritated by them?

_____

_____

_____

There is only one thing I must do this week:
Go into labor!

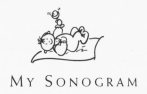

My Sonogram

[Paste sonogram here]

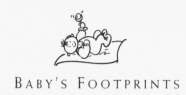

BABY'S FOOTPRINTS

[Paste baby's footprints here]

Questions to Ask a Healthcare Provider

Early on, you'll be selecting a doctor (or midwife) to take care of you during your pregnancy and to be present at the birth of your baby. Here are some questions to ask that will help you make your choice:

- ➤ *How long have you been in practice?*
- ➤ *How many babies have you delivered?*
- ➤ *What hospitals or birth centers are you affiliated with?*
- ➤ *How often will I have appointments during my pregnancy?*
- ➤ *What would cause you to see me more often than this?*
- ➤ *How much time do you set aside for each appointment?*
- ➤ *What takes place during an appointment?*
- ➤ *Will I have appointments with others in your practice?*
- ➤ *Who will deliver my baby if you're not available?*
- ➤ *Which prenatal tests do you routinely recommend?*
- ➤ *What would cause you to recommend me to the care of another health-care provider or specialist?*
- ➤ *How would I reach you in case of an emergency?*
- ➤ *How often are you on call?*
- ➤ *Do you expect to be on call around the time that my baby is due?*
- ➤ *How much time will you be able to spend with me while I'm in labor?*
- ➤ *What pain management options will I have during labor?*
- ➤ *Under what circumstances do you induce labor?*
- ➤ *Do you use electronic fetal monitoring during labor?*
- ➤ *What percentage of your patients receive episiotomies?*
- ➤ *When do you recommend a cesarean section?*
- ➤ *How often do your patients end up delivering through cesarean sections?*
- ➤ *Will my baby be able to remain with me after the birth?*
- ➤ *How often will I see you during the postpartum period?*

MEDICAL HISTORY QUESTIONS YOU WILL BE ASKED

During your first prenatal appointment, you will be asked a series of questions about your own medical history, as well as that of your baby's father and both of your families. You'll find it helpful to have the answers to the following questions ready in advance:

➤ *Do you have any chronic illnesses?*

➤ *Do you have any chronic conditions?*

➤ *What medications (prescription and over-the-counter) do you take?*

➤ *Do you take vitamins?*

➤ *Do you take herbal or dietary supplements?*

➤ *Do you have any allergies?*

➤ *Have you ever had surgery?*

➤ *What was the date of your last menstrual period?*

➤ *At what age did you start getting your period?*

➤ *How long do your periods typically last?*

➤ *How often do they occur?*

➤ *Do you have bleeding between periods?*

➤ *What kind of contraception have you used in the past year?*

➤ *Have you been tested or treated for infertility?*

➤ *How many biological children do you have?*

➤ *How old are they? What were their birth weights?*

➤ *How many times have you been pregnant?*

➤ *Were there any complications during previous pregnancies?*

➤ *Were there complications during previous deliveries?*

➤ *What types of delivery did you have during previous childbirths?*

➤ *Have you ever had a miscarriage? If so, how many?*

➤ *Have you ever had an abortion? If so, how many?*

- ➤ *Do you exercise? If so, what kind of exercise do you do? How often?*
- ➤ *Do you smoke?*
- ➤ *Do you drink alcohol?*
- ➤ *Have you ever used recreational drugs?*
- ➤ *Do you have any sexually transmitted diseases?*

- ➤ *Chronic illnesses?*
- ➤ *Chronic conditions?*
- ➤ *Allergies?*
- ➤ *History of drug or alcohol abuse?*
- ➤ *Any sexually transmitted diseases?*

FAMILY HISTORY

Is your mother living? If so, how old is she? If not, how old was she when she died? What was the cause of death? Did she suffer from any chronic health conditions or serious illnesses? How many children did your mother have? Were there any health issues during any of her pregnancies?

Is your father living? If so, how old is he? If not, how old was he when he died? What was the cause of death? Did he suffer from any chronic health conditions or serious illnesses?

How many siblings do you have? What are their ages? If any are deceased, what was the cause of death? Have any of your siblings had any chronic health conditions or serious illnesses? Have any of your sisters had health issues during pregnancy?

Was anyone in your family or in your baby's father's family born with any genetic conditions (such as cystic fibrosis, Down syndrome, Huntington's disease, etc.)?

BABY GEAR LIST

As you prepare for your baby's arrival, you'll be gathering all kinds of baby gear. Some things you'll need to buy new (the crib mattress and car seat always should be new). But before you run out and buy everything you need, wait and see what comes your way. You will receive many items as gifts; others may be cherished secondhand items that family members or friends will want to pass along to you.

The following checklist suggests basic items to have on hand:

- ❑ *Crib*
- ❑ *Crib mattress*
- ❑ *Fitted crib sheets*
- ❑ *Crib bumper*
- ❑ *Cradle*
- ❑ *Changing table*
- ❑ *Portable changing pad*
- ❑ *Baby monitor*
- ❑ *Bottles*
- ❑ *Bottle brush*
- ❑ *Nipples*
- ❑ *Nipple brush*
- ❑ *Breast pump (if you will be breastfeeding)*
- ❑ *Nursing bras*

- ❑ *Nursing nightgowns (or ones that button down the front)*
- ❑ *Bibs*
- ❑ *Sterilizer*
- ❑ *Baby bathtub*
- ❑ *Baby carriage/stroller*
- ❑ *Car seat*
- ❑ *Baby carrier/sling*
- ❑ *Diapers*
- ❑ *Diaper pail*
- ❑ *Blanket*
- ❑ *Baby toiletries (antibiotic ointment, baby wipes, diaper rash cream, medicine dropper, baby nail clippers, nasal aspirator, etc.)*
- ❑ *Baby clothes*

Shower given by _____

GIFT TRACKER/BABY SHOWER LIST

Giver	*Gift*	*Thank-You Note Sent*
_____	_____	_____
_____	_____	_____
_____	_____	_____
_____	_____	_____
_____	_____	_____
_____	_____	_____
_____	_____	_____
_____	_____	_____
_____	_____	_____
_____	_____	_____
_____	_____	_____
_____	_____	_____
_____	_____	_____
_____	_____	_____
_____	_____	_____
_____	_____	_____
_____	_____	_____
_____	_____	_____

Giver	Gift	Thank-You Note Sent
_____	_____	_____
_____	_____	_____
_____	_____	_____
_____	_____	_____
_____	_____	_____
_____	_____	_____
_____	_____	_____
_____	_____	_____
_____	_____	_____
_____	_____	_____
_____	_____	_____
_____	_____	_____
_____	_____	_____
_____	_____	_____
_____	_____	_____
_____	_____	_____
_____	_____	_____
_____	_____	_____
_____	_____	_____

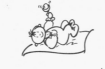

SELECTING A NAME

Choosing a name for your baby can be both challenging and fun. You and your partner may find it helpful to write down each name as it comes up, along with the der-
ivation and any special meaning for you. You'll also want to eliminate names as you
decide against them, narrowing your choices to a shorter and shorter list as you go
along.

Boys' Names

First	Middle	Meaning for You/Source
_____	_____	_____
_____	_____	_____
_____	_____	_____
_____	_____	_____
_____	_____	_____
_____	_____	_____
_____	_____	_____
_____	_____	_____
_____	_____	_____
_____	_____	_____
_____	_____	_____
_____	_____	_____
_____	_____	_____

First   Middle   Meaning for You/Source

_____ _____   _____

_____ _____   _____

_____ _____   _____

First   Middle   Meaning for You/Source

_____ _____   _____

_____ _____   _____

_____ _____   _____

_____ _____   _____

_____ _____   _____

_____ _____   _____

_____ _____   _____

_____ _____   _____

_____ _____   _____

_____ _____   _____

_____ _____   _____

_____ _____   _____

_____ _____   _____

_____ _____   _____

_____ _____   _____

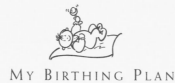

My Birthing Plan

A birthing plan can be a very detailed listing of what you want or a simple listing of your concerns and preferences about labor and delivery. You should find out what your options are and discuss what you want with your health-care giver. Remember, not everything you'll want may be available, and things don't always go according to plan—but getting your wishes down on paper now can help ease your mind a bit for later on. Here are some typical questions to consider:

➤ *Do I want to give birth in a birthing room or a delivery room?*
➤ *Who should be present at the birth?*
➤ *Do I want to walk around, sit up, or stay in bed during labor?*
➤ *Will the birth be videotaped? Who will do the taping?*
➤ *Should the lights be low?*
➤ *Are there special items from home I'll want to have with me?*
➤ *Do I want music playing while I'm in labor?*
➤ *Should a television be available?*
➤ *What position do I want to be in when I give birth?*
➤ *Might I want to have labor induced?*
➤ *Do I want medical personnel to wait for me to request pain relief or offer it before-hand?*
➤ *What kind of pain relief do I prefer? Are there any that should not be used?*
➤ *Do I want a routine episiotomy?*
➤ *Do I want to see my baby's head during the delivery?*
➤ *Should my birth partner be present if I have to have a cesarean delivery?*
➤ *Who should cut the umbilical cord?*
➤ *Do I want to hold the baby immediately after birth?*
➤ *Do I want to attempt breastfeeding right after birth?*
➤ *Will someone at the hospital be available for breastfeeding assistance?*
➤ *Can my new baby sleep in the room with me? What about my partner?*

➢ *Whom do I want to visit me in the hospital? What about children?*

➢ *How long will I stay in the hospital with a normal vaginal delivery? How about after a cesarean section?*

➢ *Do I have any other important concerns, questions, or preferences?*

_____

_____

_____

_____

_____

_____

_____

_____

_____

_____

Packing for the Hospital

You'll want to have everything possible packed and ready for the big day. That way, you, or, more likely, your partner, won't have to run around looking for specific items at the last minute.

Before you even pack your bag, you should know the best route to the hospital (plus more than one alternative), which hospital entrance to use, and where to report in. Have on hand the telephone numbers for your local cab company, the ambulance service, and a friend, relative, or neighbor who can drive you in a pinch.

The following items can be assembled in advance:

- ❑ *Identification*
- ❑ *Insurance card*
- ❑ *Preregistration forms*
- ❑ *List of names to call*
- ❑ *Copy of birthing plan*
- ❑ *2 nursing bras (if you intend to breastfeed)*
- ❑ *Nightgown or pajamas (button-down if you intend to breastfeed)*
- ❑ *Robe*
- ❑ *Slippers*
- ❑ *Warm socks*
- ❑ *Several pairs of underwear*
- ❑ *Hairbrush*
- ❑ *Shampoo and conditioner*
- ❑ *Toothpaste and toothbrush*
- ❑ *Soap*
- ❑ *Washcloths and towels*
- ❑ *Shower slippers*
- ❑ *Watch with a second hand (for timing contractions)*
- ❑ *Camera or video camera*

- ❑ *Going-home outfit*
- ❑ *Tissues*
- ❑ *Hot water bottle*
- ❑ *Lip balm*
- ❑ *Body lotion*
- ❑ *Several highly absorbent sanitary napkins*
- ❑ *Snacks for you and your partner*
- ❑ *CDs and CD player*
- ❑ *Magazines*
- ❑ *A cell phone (or a roll of quarters or prepaid phone card)*
- ❑ *Tennis ball or rolling pin to massage your back during labor*

- ❑ *3-4 undershirts and onesies*
- ❑ *Special outfit and cap to wear home*
- ❑ *Receiving blanket*
- ❑ *Warm coat and hat, if it's cold*
- ❑ *Car seat*

_____

_____

_____

_____

_____

_____

_____

_____

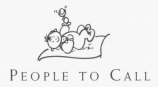

PEOPLE TO CALL

There are lots of people to call when your baby is about to be born. You must first inform all the key people who will be involved in the delivery and birth. Of course, you'll want to call some special friends and family members when you go into labor. Others you or your partner can call after you have given birth. But having all these numbers available on one sheet of paper will save a lot of time and energy.

Spouse/partner (if not with you when you go into labor) _____

Health-care provider _____

Hospital _____

Birth coach _____

Midwife or doula _____

Baby-sitter for your children _____

Parents (yours and your partner's) _____

_____

_____

Siblings (yours and your partner's) _____

_____

_____

*Other family*_____

_____

_____

Close friends _____

_____

_____

*Your employer*_____

Coworkers (Hint: If you designate one coworker to call or e-mail, that person can spread the word to everyone else at work.) _____

_____

LABOR RECORD

My labor started on _____ at _____

I went into the hospital on _____ at _____

How I felt when I arrived at the hospital _____

_____

_____

I was in labor for _____ hours and _____ minutes

What pain relief did I use? _____

Who was present at the birth? _____

_____

_____

Who cut the umbilical cord? _____

Did the baby cry immediately? _____

Was childbirth what I imagined it would be? _____

_____

_____

How was it different? _____

_____

_____

What would I do differently? _____

_____

_____

_____

How do I feel now that my baby has been born? _____

_____

_____

_____

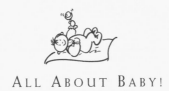

ALL ABOUT BABY!

Name: _____

Date of birth: _____

Time of birth: _____

Weight: _____

Length: _____

Apgar score: _____

Comments: _____

_____

_____

_____

_____

_____

_____

_____

_____

WHAT HAPPENED ON THE DAY MY BABY WAS BORN?

What was the weather like on the day my baby was born? _____

_____

What local, national, or world events were in the news the day my baby was born?

Local: _____

_____

_____

National: _____

_____

_____

World events: _____

_____

_____

What important events happened on this date in history?

_____

_____

_____

_____

_____

_____

_____

Questions to Ask When Leaving the Hospital

Before you leave the hospital, you should have the answers to certain basic questions about your baby and yourself. Here's what you'll need to know:

Caring for the Baby

➤ What feeding schedule should the baby be on?

➤ What kind of bathing routine should I use?

➤ What should I do if the baby is crying? Do different kinds of crying indicate different things?

➤ What about umbilical cord care?

➤ What is a normal sleep pattern for a newborn? What might indicate a problem?

➤ How do I care for a boy's circumcision?

➤ Are there any other important instructions?

➤ When should I call for baby's first well-baby visit?

Caring for Yourself

➤ Are there any activities I need to avoid and, if so, for how long?

➤ Is it okay for me to drive?

➤ Can I resume exercising? If so, what kind of exercises?

➤ When will my stitches be healed? How should I care for my stitches?

➤ Can I take hot baths?

➤ Do I need to do anything special to care for my episiotomy site and/or hemorrhoids?

➤ What do I need to know about recovering from a cesarean section (if applicable)?

➤ Do you have any tips on coping with breast engorgement or nipple soreness?

➤ Who can I call if I have breastfeeding questions or issues?

➤ Are there any foods or medications to avoid if I plan to breastfeed?

➤ Can I resume sexual activity?

➤ When should I start using birth control? Can you recommend birth control options?

Maternal and Child Health Bureau
(U.S. Department of Health and Human Services)
18-05 Parklawn Building
5600 Fishers Lane
Rockville, MD 20857
301-443-2170
www.mchb.hrsa.gov

National Women's Health Network
514 10th Street, NW
Suite 400
Washington, D.C. 20004
202-347-1140
www.womenshealthnetwork.org

Other Helpful Websites
www.ssa.gov/OACT/babynames/—The Social Security Administration's online
name-tracking search engine
www.babycenter.com
www.childbirth.org
www.familyweb.com
www.parentingweb.com

_____

_____

_____

_____

_____

_____

_____

_____

_____

BABY'S FIRST PHOTO

[Paste baby's first photo here]

Moments and Milestones
Pregnancy Journal
A Week-by-Week Companion

Jennifer Leigh Youngs and Bettie B. Youngs, Ph.D., Ed.D.

Need more gifts for expectant moms? Save a bundle by ordering multiple copies at a special discount! For details, contact the AMACOM Books Special Sales Department at

Tel.: 212-903-8316

Fax: 212-903-8083

Website: www.amacombooks.org/special

ISBN-10: 0-8144-7377-6
ISBN-13: 978-0-8144-7377-1

Interior book design: DesignPlus, Koehli/LeBrun

Printing number

10 9 8 7 6 5 4 3 2 1